DIY
BEAUTY

Easy, All-Natural Recipes Based on Your Favorites
from **Lush**, **Kiehl's**, **Burt's Bees**, **Bumble and bumble**,
Laura Mercier, and More!

INA DE CLERCQ

Adams Media

New York   London   Toronto   Sydney   New Delhi

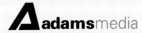

Adams Media
An Imprint of Simon & Schuster, Inc.
57 Littlefield Street
Avon, Massachusetts 02322

First Adams Media hardcover edition June 2019

ADAMS MEDIA and colophon are trademarks of Simon & Schuster.

For information about special discounts for bulk purchases, please contact Simon & Schuster Special Sales at 1-866-506-1949 or business@simonandschuster.com.

The Simon & Schuster Speakers Bureau can bring authors to your live event. For more information or to book an event contact the Simon & Schuster Speakers Bureau at 1-866-248-3049 or visit our website at www.simonspeakers .com.

Interior design by Sylvia McArdle
Interior images by Harper Point Photography

Manufactured in the United States of America

10 9 8 7 6 5 4 3 2 1

Library of Congress Cataloging-in-Publication Data
Names: De Clercq, Ina, author.
Title: DIY beauty / Ina De Clercq.
Description: Avon, Massachusetts: Adams Media, 2019.
Includes index.
Identifiers: LCCN 2018055722 | ISBN 9781507209424 (hc) | ISBN 9781507209431 (ebook)
Subjects: LCSH: Beauty, Personal. | Cosmetics. | Handicraft.
Classification: LCC RA778 .D2855 2019 | DDC 646.7/2--dc23
LC record available at https://lccn.loc.gov/2018055722

ISBN 978-1-5072-0942-4
ISBN 978-1-5072-0943-1 (ebook)

ACKNOWLEDGMENTS

Thank you to my readers for following my adventures both online and now offline.

Thanks to Julia, Brett, and the entire team at Simon & Schuster for bringing this book to life.

Thank you to the School of Natural Skincare for contributing to my insights in making my own skincare products. The school has been a great resource for me during my DIY journey. I highly recommend their online courses if you want to take the next step in your own journey with homemade beauty products.

Thanks to Jeroen for seeing opportunities I can't and believing in me when I don't.

And thanks to Mono, my cat, for being my emotional support system. Even if she's blissfully unaware of it.

REFERENCE

Special thanks to the School of Natural Skincare and its course Certificate in Making Natural Skincare Products. I highly recommend their courses if you want to continue your journey in making your own homemade beauty products.

CONTENTS

CHAPTER 3

SHINE THERAPY 52

CHAPTER 6
BATH FUN . . . 144

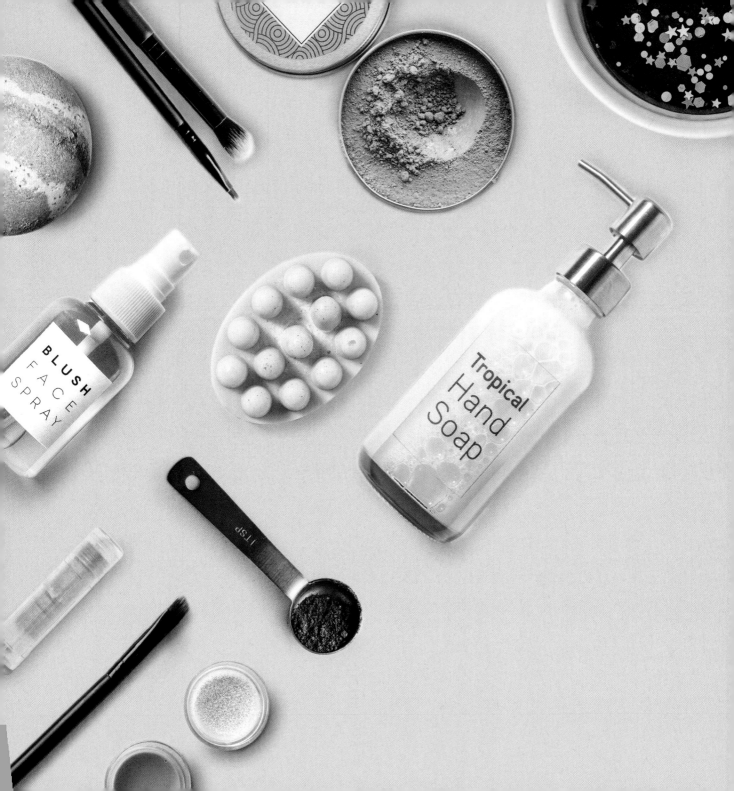

INTRODUCTION

Love Lush?
Can't stop shopping at Sephora?
Need a whole closet for all your Bath & Body Works products?

If you can't get enough of your favorite beauty supplies but wish you could find less expensive and more natural versions of them, then you should try making your own beauty products!

Making your own beauty supplies is easier, faster, and more fun than you might imagine, and it gives you the same level of quality you can find in store-bought products without all the unnecessary (and sometimes harmful) chemicals and additives.

With *DIY Beauty*, you can make customized versions of the beauty products you love using simple and natural ingredients. Inside you'll find recipes to make your own:

• Face masks • Lip balms • Eye masks • Hair treatments • Makeup powders • Bath bombs • Body creams • and more!

The one hundred beauty recipes in *DIY Beauty* are inspired by top brands and products and will help you make your own skincare staples at home, from "whatever-is-in-your-fridge" face masks to luxurious soap and lotion bars. Once you try making your own beauty products, you'll discover that it's easy, doesn't break the bank, and leaves your skin looking and feeling better than ever before.

Are you ready to take control of your beauty routine and get the glowing and beautiful skin you always dreamed of? Then let's go!

1

CHAPTER 1

READY. SET. SHINE!

The goal of this book is to show you that you can take control of your beauty routine by making your own skincare remedies with just a few simple, all-natural ingredients. In this first chapter you'll find everything you need to get started. You'll learn how to prep your workspace, what materials you need to make your own beauty products, and what techniques you'll have to master. You'll also learn more about all those wonderful natural ingredients and their benefits for your skin, including my favorite basic ingredients that we'll be using a lot in the recipes of this book.

THE BEAUTY OF DIY BEAUTY

There are many reasons why you might want to make your own face masks, body butters, bath bombs, or lip balms. Maybe your eye fell on the ingredients list of your favorite beauty product one day and you were surprised to find that you couldn't pronounce any of them. Maybe your skin reacts badly to certain products, even those that claim to be hypoallergenic. Or maybe you just really like to DIY. Whatever your reasons, you'll find there are many benefits to making your own beauty products, including these:

You Know Exactly What Is in Your Products

Natural ingredients are all the rage right now, and more and more brands boast about using certain natural ingredients. But when you look at the actual ingredient list of the product, you might find these ingredients all the way down at the bottom of the list. That might mean the amount used is actually tiny. Sometimes it accounts for only 1 percent or less of the final product. If a recipe in this book says it uses the power of green tea, for example, you can be sure it's one of the main ingredients in the recipe.

...and What Isn't in Them

If you know exactly what goes into a beauty product, you can make sure the ingredients are only the best for your skin. A lot of people are allergic or sensitive to the unnecessary fragrances and colorants that are added to many beauty products. The recipes in this book keep it simple and don't require anything other than ingredients that are meant to help your skin.

The recipes in this book aren't identical to the products that inspired them. How could they be? We are using only a few simple, all-natural ingredients. No fillers, no synthetic ingredients, and no preservatives. The recipes in this book do use similar ingredients and/or are intended to have a similar effect on your skin. This book will show you that with just a few simple ingredients, you can become your own skincare developer.

PREP YOUR SPACE

A lot of effort and love go into making your homemade beauty products. And it all starts with a clean workspace. This might seem obvious, but it's a crucial part of making your own skincare products. After all, when you're cooking dinner or baking a cake, you make sure you work in a clean environment. You don't want anything ending up in your cake that doesn't belong there, do you? The same goes for when you're crafting your own beauty products. Follow these rules when prepping your workspace:

- **Start with a clean slate.** Make sure you thoroughly clean your workspace and surfaces before you begin.

- **Use clean materials.** To clean my materials, I use my dishwasher. If you go this route, make sure your dishwasher is in good condition and your equipment comes out clean and dry! You can also use 70 percent isopropyl alcohol or sterilizing fluid to further sanitize your materials.

- **Help prevent spills and stains.** Cover workspaces to keep them safe from spilling, and be especially careful when you're using waxes and essential oils, which can make a mess.

- **Keep yourself clean too!** Always wash your hands before you begin. You can also wear an apron and gloves to protect yourself, and a hair net to keep your products clean.

Your DIY Beauty Tool Kit

Now that your work area is prepped and ready to go, it's time to gather your materials. Here are some of the materials you'll need for making your beauty creations:

- **Measuring cups and spoons:** Some of the recipes in this book use teaspoons, tablespoons, and cups as measurements for dry ingredients or small quantities. Regular kitchen spoons come in many shapes and sizes, so I recommend investing in a good set of measuring cups and spoons. Choose high-quality stainless steel, glass, or ceramic tools. Also, when making the products in this book, don't add heaping spoon- or cupfuls. Make sure the ingredient is level with the edges of the spoon or cup unless otherwise specified.

- **Kitchen scale:** Many of the ingredients in this book are measured in ounces, so you need a kitchen scale to make sure these measurements are precise.

- **Heatproof mixing bowls:** To combine your ingredients you'll need mixing bowls. Make sure they are heatproof, as they'll be handling melted waxes, butters, and oils.

There's no better gift than one that's handmade with love. Whether you've been making your own gifts for years or you're more of a ready-made kind of gal/guy, in this book you'll find plenty of DIY ideas—not just to make for yourself but to hand out to friends and family as well. Homemade bath bombs really do make the best holiday and birthday gifts!

- **Spoons, spatulas, or hand whisks:** To mix the ingredients together you can use regular spoons, spatulas, or hand whisks—or even single-use chopsticks.

- **Electric whisk or mixer:** To give body butters their creamy consistency you need to whip them into shape. Find an electric whisk or mixer that can be adjusted to a low setting, or you'll have bits of lotion flying everywhere. I use a food processor with a whisk attachment, and it is the *best* lotion whipper!

- **High-speed blender:** With a blender you can turn food items and face mask ingredients into "smoothies" for your face.

- **Microwave:** If a recipe calls for a melted butter or oil, you can quickly melt it in your microwave. If you don't own a microwave, use the double boiler method instead.

- **Double boiler:** The double boiler method is considered the easiest, most professional way to melt your natural waxes, butters, and oils together. If you've never heard of this technique, read more in the next section.

It's important that you make sure no water gets into the top pan of your double boiler. Why? I'll explain why water is your frenemy in Chapter 2.

The Double Boiler (So Important It Needs Its Own Section!)

You might have heard the double boiler method referred to as a water bath or bain-marie. If you've never used this method, it might sound like a very complicated technique, but I can assure you it really isn't.

First, you'll fill a medium saucepan about halfway with water. Place the saucepan on your stove over medium heat. Let the water heat up until it's nearly boiling. Then adjust the heat underneath until the water is lightly simmering.

Then place a smaller saucepan on top of the first saucepan. The bottom of the smaller pan should be submerged by the water about 1 inch. Let the handles of the smaller pan rest on the sides of the pan underneath. You can also use a double boiler insert (sometimes called a melting pot) for this. This top saucepan or melting pot will be where you'll put your waxes and butter.

The purpose of the double boiler is to gently melt ingredients so they do not overheat, scorch, or burn. This method provides you with slow and even heat. Keep in mind that both pans will get hot, so use pot holders or a towel when touching or moving the pans. Feel free to lower the heat if you need to; as long as the ingredients are melting, you're good.

DIY BEAUTY SHOPPING LIST

It's time to go shopping! Some of the ingredients in this book are common grocery items, like Greek yogurt and strawberries, and some are kitchen staples, like baking soda. But if you really want to get serious about DIY beauty, you have to get to know your waxes, butters, and oils. You will see that these ingredients appear in a lot of the recipes in this book. Changing something as simple as the ratio can take the same ingredients from a lip balm to a cleansing balm. Every ingredient in this list is used in more than one recipe. So when you buy a new ingredient for your stash, you know you will put it to good use. Here are some of the items you will need to purchase for the recipes in this book:

Beeswax

There are many kinds of waxes that are suitable for cosmetic use, but beeswax is by far the most common. Beeswax creates a barrier that slows the loss of water from your skin. And that's pretty awesome, because it keeps your skin hydrated and moisturized.

You can find beeswax in bar or pellet form in online stores. It all comes down to your preference, but I find pellets easier to measure when making beauty products. Beeswax typically has a golden hue, but you can also buy naturally filtered white beeswax. This is a great choice if you want to add your own color to a product, like an eye shadow or a tinted lip balm.

If you're looking for a vegan option, there are some alternatives you can use instead. These include candelilla wax, carnauba wax, and Japan wax. Every wax has its own level of hardness, so you will have to experiment with the ratios in the recipe if you decide to swap.

Butters

If you've just started making your own beauty products, shea butter and cocoa butter will probably be your go-to choices. But don't overlook some of the other amazing butters, like mango and avocado butter. Both avocado and mango butter feel drier on the skin than shea butter, so you can swap them in body balm recipes for a less greasy feel.

You can find refined and unrefined butters. Most of the time unrefined butters are preferred for beauty products.

Plant-Based Oils

For years we've been told that oils are bad. Who would ever think to put an oil on oily skin? Well, I would, because for me oils were the hack to a perfectly balanced, shine-free skin. Oils from nuts, seeds, or plants are an important ingredient in many natural skincare products. You might know them as carrier oils. These oils are rich in essential fatty acids, minerals, and vitamins that help your skin look and feel great. Refer to Chapter 3 for an overview of my favorite carrier oils.

Cosmetic Mica

I can't get enough of glitter. But I'm not a fan of the plastic it's made of. Enter mica. Mica is a naturally occurring mineral found in rocks. It's used to add color and sparkle to many things, including cosmetic products.

Mica comes in many colors, from bright, bold hues to a shimmery pearl or gold. As the mica you buy for your beauty products should be approved for cosmetic use, I refer to it in the recipes in this book as cosmetic mica. Check carefully before you buy it to see if it can be used on your skin and especially on your face, for example in lip and eye products.

Citric Acid

You'll see this ingredient a lot in Chapter 6, the Bath Fun chapter. Don't let the term *acid* scare you. Citric acid is a natural compound found in fruits like oranges and lemons. The citric acid powder you can buy in bulk is a very concentrated form of this natural compound. It's often used as a natural preservative in foods, but I like it best for making bath bombs. With a 1-pound bag you can make about sixteen regular-sized bath bombs. Give it a try and order a bag online. I bet you'll be ordering it on repeat.

ABOUT ESSENTIAL OILS

Essential oils are a great addition to your homemade beauty products. In fact, you'll find them in a large majority of the recipes in this book. However, there are also some precautions you need to take when working with and using essential oils. If you want to enjoy the amazing benefits of essential oils in your homemade skincare products, there are a few must-follow guidelines.

Patch Test First

When making your own beauty products, it's good to keep in mind that anyone can have an allergic or sensitive reaction to anything at any time. I even know a girl who's allergic to chocolate! Since essential oils are highly concentrated, it's recommended to perform a patch test with them first.

One way to do a patch test is by diluting one drop of essential oil in 0.2 ounce of carrier oil (this can be olive oil or another carrier oil of your choice). Apply a little bit of the mixture to the inside of your elbow and wait 24 hours to see if a reaction occurs. If so, don't use the product on your skin!

If you're making a product with essential oils for a friend, tell them to do a patch test with the product before use and ask them if they've previously had an allergic reaction to essential oils (or any of the other ingredients). As always, it's better to be safe than sorry.

Essential oils don't dissolve in water, so don't scatter those drops directly into your bathwater. Dilute them first in a carrier oil or use bath salts instead. Check out Chapter 6 for some great recipe ideas!

Less Really Is More

Always dilute your essential oils in a carrier oil. For each recipe in this book that includes essential oils, I've listed a recommended amount. But feel free to use fewer drops than the recipe calls for. The tolerance for an essential oil can vary from one person to the next.

Always Read the Label

If you buy your ingredients from a high-quality brand, the label should give you useful information, like guidelines for safe use and storage. Some essential oils are not recommended when you're pregnant, some require specific dilution rates, and so on. All of this information should be mentioned on the package or on the bottle. Always follow the restrictions and contraindications provided by the brand. They know their products best!

Don't Underestimate Their Power

Essential oils are the goodness of a plant or flower captured in a tiny bottle. That also means essential oils are highly concentrated. A little goes a long way when it comes to including essential oils in your DIY beauty skincare routine.

Irritation of the skin can occur if you don't use the appropriate ratio of essential oil. When this happens, your skin will look red and sting or burn. For instant relief, gently rub a small amount of plant-based oil onto the area. Wipe clean with a piece of cloth. Repeat as often as necessary. Check with your doctor if the irritation doesn't go away.

Before You Buy

When shopping for essential oils you'll notice that there's a big price range, from pricey rosa damascena to the more common lavender essential oil. Don't let that hefty price tag scare you. You need only a tiny amount each time you make a beauty product. I recommend starting your collection with a few multipurpose essential oils. Check my guide in Chapter 4 for my favorite starter picks!

Homemade skincare products, just like store-bought products, are never meant to sting, hurt, or burn. Everybody's skin is different and can react differently to certain products and ingredients. A product that works great for you could be too strong for someone else. If you're allergic to a food item, then don't use it in a skincare product either. If you're allergic to almonds, for example, you can swap sweet almond oil for another carrier oil, like olive oil.

It's always a good idea to perform a patch test before using a product. Use a small amount of the product on a small patch of skin, on your arm, for example. Wait 24 hours to see if a reaction occurs.

Since you're investing in an essential oil, make sure you go for high quality. A high-quality essential oil will be sold in a dark amber or blue glass bottle and will include information for safe use.

How to Store Essential Oils

Now that you've started your own collection of essential oils, you'll need to store them somewhere safe so you get the most bang for your buck. As with all your ingredients, remember to keep them in a cool, dry, and dark place out of direct sunlight. Oh, and out of reach of children and pets, of course. Make sure you place the caps back onto the right bottles after each use, and make sure they are screwed on tight to avoid accidents.

WHERE TO SHOP

So now that you know some of the ingredients you'll need to buy to make your own beauty products, you may be wondering where you can buy them. Here are some options:

- **Grocery store or farmers' market:** You can get good-quality, organic ingredients from your local farmers' market or grocery store. Food items like coconut milk and cucumber can easily be found here. Some ingredients, like strawberries, might not be available all year round. Citric acid can typically be found in the canning aisle of larger supermarkets. Agar agar powder should be in the baking aisle. You can always ask for help if you can't find an ingredient right away. Also, don't be afraid to think outside the box when shopping for your ingredients. Does your farmers' market have a honey stand? Ask the beekeeper if he or she sells beeswax too!

- **Drugstore, health store, or pharmacy:** You might be surprised by what you can find at your local drugstore, health store, or pharmacy. Activated charcoal capsules, aloe vera gel, and bentonite clay can commonly be found on the shelves at these establishments. Some sell a good range of basic carrier oils, too, like jojoba oil and sweet almond oil. Be critical before you buy, and read those labels. Go for pure, good-quality ingredients.

- **Online retailers:** You can find and order less common ingredients, like waxes, butters, oils, and clays, online from different web stores. Check the reviews and carefully read the product descriptions before making your purchase.

Choose good-quality ingredients for your DIY beauty products. Make sure that they are labeled for cosmetic use, and don't forget to check their expiration dates.

Also, don't let the price influence you too much. A 2-ounce bottle or an 8-pound bag makes *a lot* of beauty products. With a 4-ounce container of shea butter, for example, you can make at least one body butter, a cleansing balm, two solid eye shadows, and eight lip balms following the recipes in this book.

SAFE STORAGE

Once you've made your beauty products, you want them to last as long as possible. Here are some tips to help with that:

- Store your homemade beauty products in clean, dry, and dark airtight containers. I'm all for zero waste, so it's great if you can reuse your containers. Just make sure you thoroughly clean and sterilize them before each use.

- Store your ingredients and homemade products in a cool, dry, and dark place. Keep them out of direct sunlight, as exposure to light will speed up the oxidization of the butters and oils.

- Unless the instructions from a recipe say otherwise, the oil-based products you make will be at their best at room temperature. Store them tightly sealed in the refrigerator on hot summer days.

- Water-based products should always be kept in the refrigerator.

The recipes in this book keep it simple and are made without preservatives. Because of that there's always a risk that your products could become contaminated. Read more about what to look out for in Chapter 2.

Each recipe in this book comes with an indication for how long the product can keep. These are estimations based on general guidelines and my own personal experience. There are a lot of variables that come into play when determining the shelf life of a product. There are the conditions in which the product is made, the expiration date of each individual ingredient, and so on. As a general rule we're using 6 months as the final expiration date for oil-based products, and 3 months if we're using oils with a shorter shelf life. Water-based products are an entirely different story. Even if you use a flower water or aloe vera gel that contains preservatives, we're adding other ingredients to it and making an entirely new product. Use these products only right after you've made them. It's better to be safe than sorry!

PERFECT PACKAGING

Whether you are making these DIY beauty products for yourself or as presents for others, there's no reason why you can't have a bit of fun with your packaging. Visit your local craft store or beauty supply company to find storage containers and packages ranging from the practical to the unique. Depending on what you make, you may need pump bottles, jars, tins, tubes, or bottles. Here are some packaging suggestions:

- Clear glass or plastic bottles allow you to see the contents, which is lovely if you're using infused herbs and other vibrant ingredients. Just be sure to store products in clear containers in a cool, dark place.

- Dark amber or blue glass bottles are also attractive and will protect your products longer.

- If you're giving away your bath bombs as gifts, try wrapping them in colored tissue paper and then in a paper gift bag or box.

- Homemade soaps look amazing wrapped in some craft paper and tied with twine and some dried flowers.

- You'll want to label your homemade products with the name of the product and other useful information. Look for fun stickers and labels online or at craft stores, and practice your creative hand-lettering skills to make your labels really pop.

- You can also make your own unique and professional-looking labels for your products online using sites like Vistaprint, StickerYou, and Labeley.com, among others.

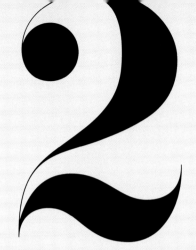

CHAPTER 2

FRESH FACED

Face masks are perfect when you're a first-time beauty DIYer. They are easy to make, and you need only a few simple ingredients that are probably already sitting in your kitchen!

My first adventure in DIY beauty was a simple oatmeal scrub. After a horrible allergic breakout on my face, I didn't feel comfortable using my store-bought cleanser anymore. So I turned to a natural remedy I had read about. When I rinsed the oatmeal mush off my skin, I was shocked. The redness from the rash was visibly reduced, and my face felt clean and balanced. I was hooked from that point on.

You don't need lots of fancy ingredients to start your own DIY beauty journey. Start by using a homemade face mask once a week or every two weeks. Invite a couple of friends over, head to the kitchen, and flip through the recipes in this chapter. I'm sure you'll fall in love with DIY face masks too.

Storage Guidelines and Tips

You'll notice that some of the recipes in this book can last all the way up to 6 months, and others should be used up right away. The main reason for this difference is water.

Preservatives have gotten a really bad rap in recent years. Not every preservative is the same, however, and most are very effective at keeping bacteria and other causes of spoiling away. You may have your own reasons for avoiding preservatives: maybe your skin is sensitive to a lot of them, or you want to keep your DIY beauty products as simple and natural as possible. Fear not; it is possible to make your own beauty products without preservatives. It just means that your homemade products will come with their own set of rules.

Without a broad-spectrum preservative there's always a risk of contamination. Icky things like bacteria and mold can grow in products that aren't kept properly and are unfortunately unavoidable over time. Follow these important guidelines to get the most out of your DIY beauty products:

- **Keep all water as far away from your products as possible!** Oil-based products don't need a preservative. But that changes as soon as you introduce water or water-based products into them. That includes aloe vera gel, honey, and flower waters. Don't store products like body scrubs and body butters in your shower. Scoop a bit of product into a separate container and take that with you. Store your products in airtight containers to keep them safe from humidity and other contaminants. (Some of the recipes in this book use water-based ingredients. As a result, you'll notice that they have a much shorter shelf life and should be stored in the refrigerator.)

- **Oils and butters can oxidize over time and go bad.** Not even a preservative can stop this process. Check the expiration dates on your ingredients. If one of the ingredients is about to expire, so is your product. The ingredient with the shortest shelf life indicates the shelf life of your final product. If this is 2 months, for example, use your homemade product within 2 months.

- **Store out of direct sunlight.** Light speeds up the oxidization process, which is why you need to keep your products out of direct sunlight and store them in dark (preferably amber or blue) containers. Adding a small percentage of vitamin E oil can also slow down that oxidization process. Read more about this oil in Chapter 3.

- **Watch out for changes in color, texture, and smell.** Any funky business—like spots appearing—should trigger alarm bells. If you have even the tiniest doubt, just throw away the product and make a fresh batch.

Treat your products with care. Only if you treat *them* well will they be able to take care of you in the best possible way!

Also, remember to write down both the date when you made the product and the estimated expiration date on the packaging. It's easy to forget after a few weeks!

CHEAT SHEET MASK

Inspired by Dr. Jart+'s Pore Minimalist Black Charcoal Sheet Mask

MAKES 1 FACE MASK

1 capsule activated charcoal

½ teaspoon Moroccan lava clay

1 tablespoon water

1 cotton sheet mask

This feisty detox mask will draw impurities from your pores, revealing tingly, fresh skin.

HOW TO MAKE:

1 Carefully open activated charcoal capsule and pour powder into a small mixing bowl.

2 Add Moroccan lava clay and water. Stir well to combine.

3 Pour the mixture onto a large plate and spread out evenly. Place the sheet mask on top and leave it at least 5 minutes or until the mask has soaked up all the liquid.

HOW TO USE:

1 Make sure your face is clean and dry. Apply the mask to your face and pat it down with your fingertips. Let the mask sit 5–10 minutes.

2 Remove the mask and rinse your face thoroughly with water.

3 Follow with a mild toner or flower water to remove every trace of the face mask.

HOW TO STORE:

This face mask is meant for a single, immediate use. You can mix the dry ingredients and keep them in an airtight container up to 6 months. When you're ready to mix your mask, scoop the amount you need out of the container into a separate mixing bowl and add water.

CLAY CLEANSER MASK

Inspired by Kiehl's Rare Earth Deep Pore Cleansing Masque

This creamy cleanser gives you the best of both worlds. The shea butter and jojoba oil cleanse and moisturize, while the clays draw impurities from your skin.

MAKES 1 (2.3-OUNCE) FACE MASK BALM

1.5 ounces shea butter

0.8 ounce jojoba oil

2 tablespoons kaolin clay

½ tablespoon bentonite clay

1 (3-ounce) airtight container

HOW TO MAKE:

1 Melt shea butter in a double boiler over medium heat. Or melt shea butter in a heatproof container in the microwave on a low setting (650 watts or lower) using 1-minute intervals until shea butter has melted.

2 Take the double boiler off the heat or take the container out of the microwave. Pour melted shea butter into a large mixing bowl. Stir in jojoba oil.

3 Cover the mixing bowl and place it in the refrigerator for about 50 minutes so that the mixture can thicken. Take it out before the mixture starts to harden.

4 Add kaolin clay and bentonite clay to the mixture. Use an electric whisk or mixer to carefully whip the ingredients into a balm. Use a low setting to prevent bits of balm from flying around. Keep whipping the mixture until it has a buttery consistency.

5 Scoop the whipped balm into the airtight container.

HOW TO USE:

1 Scoop about ½ teaspoon out of the container with clean, dry fingers or a spatula.

2 Rub the balm between your hands to melt the mixture. Massage the balm on a clean face with your fingertips.

3 Let the mask sit for a few minutes before using a warm, damp washcloth to wipe the balm from your face.

HOW TO STORE:

Store in a cool, dry place out of direct sunlight up to 3 months.

MATCHA POWER FACE MASK

Inspired by Origins' RitualiTea Matcha Madness Revitalizing Powder Face Mask

MAKES 0.6 OUNCE FACE MASK POWDER (ABOUT 10 APPLICATIONS)

3 tablespoons finely ground (colloidal) oatmeal

1 tablespoon matcha tea powder

1 (1-ounce) airtight container

This tea-shop regular will become your new go-to face mask! Matcha is rich in antioxidants, and the oatmeal grains will gently exfoliate your skin.

HOW TO MAKE:

1 Combine oatmeal and matcha powder in the airtight container.

2 Put on the lid and shake until powder has an even green color. Wait for the powder to settle at the bottom before opening the container.

2 Apply an even layer on clean, dry skin. Let it sit about 10 minutes and then rinse it off with lukewarm water.

3 Follow with a mild toner or flower water to remove every bit of the green mask.

HOW TO USE:

1 Scoop 1 heaping teaspoon face mask powder into a small mixing bowl or onto a small plate. Add 1 teaspoon water or milk. For a moisturizing boost add a drop of your favorite carrier oil, like sweet almond oil. Stir to combine all the ingredients.

HOW TO STORE:

Store in a cool, dry place and keep all water out of the container. This face mask powder can last up to 6 months. Once you've mixed the powder with the wet ingredients, you should use it all in one go.

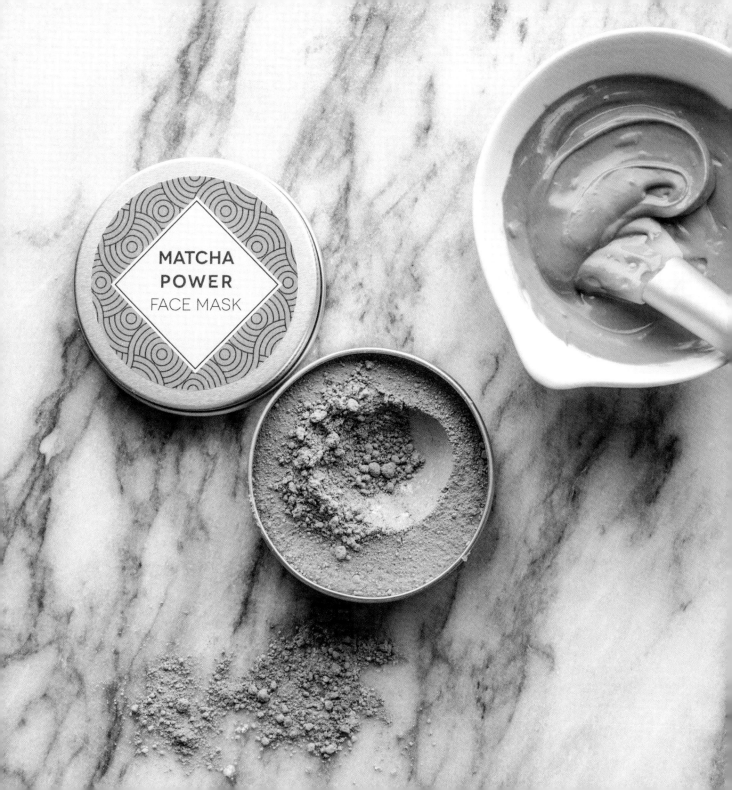

COOL DOWN MASK

Inspired by Korres's After Sun Greek Yoghurt Cooling Gel for Face & Body

MAKES 1 FACE MASK

1 tablespoon plain Greek yogurt

1 tablespoon sweet almond oil

1 tablespoon aloe vera gel

We all know by now that it's best to avoid a sunburn altogether. But just in case you get caught by surprise, here's a face mask that'll make your face feel as cool as a breeze. Use yogurt straight from the refrigerator for that extra cooling factor.

HOW TO MAKE:

Combine Greek yogurt, sweet almond oil, and aloe vera gel in a small mixing bowl. Stir together until the ingredients form a paste.

HOW TO USE:

1 Apply a thick layer all over your face and let it sit 10–20 minutes.

2 Rinse with water. This mask can be applied on other parts of the body, too, like your shoulders, back, or legs.

HOW TO STORE:

This face mask is meant for a single, immediate use.

CHIA PUDDING FACE MASK

Inspired by Dior's Hydra Life Glow Better—Fresh Jelly Mask

This chia seed pudding looks good enough to eat (and you could!). But we're using this superfood face mask to exfoliate dead skin cells and reveal fresh new skin underneath.

MAKES 1 FACE MASK

½ medium orange

1 teaspoon chia seeds

1 teaspoon maple syrup

HOW TO MAKE:

1 Squeeze 1 tablespoon juice from the orange in a small mixing bowl.

2 Add chia seeds and maple syrup. Stir the ingredients together until the seeds are evenly distributed.

3 Place the mixture in the refrigerator and let it set at least 15 minutes.

HOW TO USE:

1 Apply an even layer on clean, dry skin. Gently massage your face with your fingertips.

2 Rinse it off with plenty of water.

HOW TO STORE:

This food-based face mask is meant for a single, immediate use.

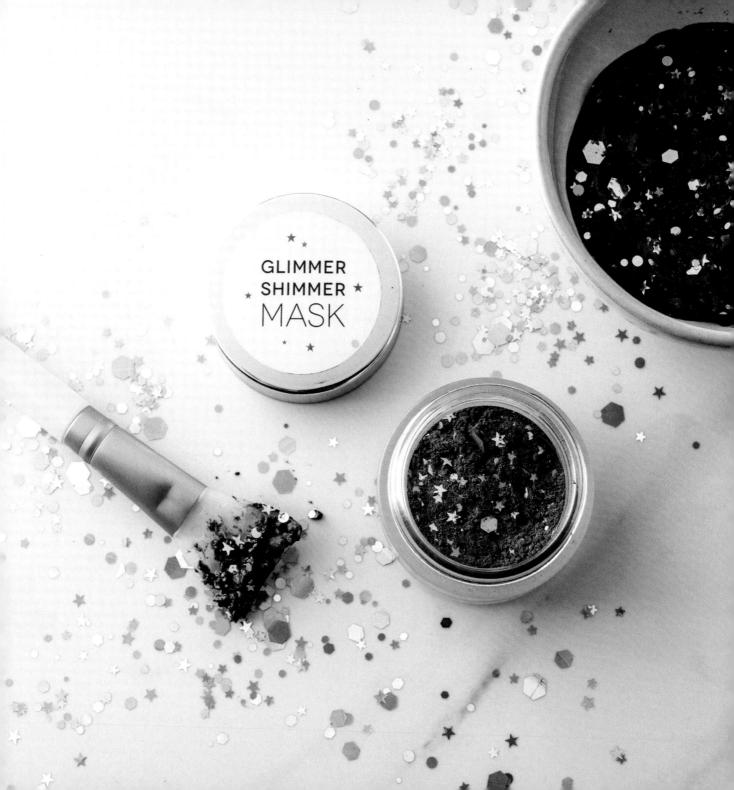

GLIMMER SHIMMER MASK

Inspired by Glamglow's #Glittermask Gravitymud

This mask glimmers with the help of glitter! However, most commercial glitter is made from plastic, which is not the best for your skin or drain! Try glitter made from a biodegradable source, such as plant materials. Edible glitter or luster dust powder is what you'd use on top of a cake or cupcake and can easily be found in the baking aisle. And jojoba beads are made from jojoba oil. These are all much better alternatives to wash down your drain!

MAKES 0.5 OUNCE FACE MASK POWDER (ABOUT 10 APPLICATIONS)

2 tablespoons marshmallow root (or rolled oats)

1 tablespoon kaolin clay

1 tablespoon agar agar powder

½ tablespoon luster dust powder or cosmetic mica

1 teaspoon biodegradable glitter or jojoba beads (optional)

1 (1-ounce) airtight container

HOW TO MAKE:

1 Grind marshmallow root or rolled oats to a fine powder in a clean coffee grinder or food processor.

2 Scoop marshmallow root powder or oat powder into a small mixing bowl and add kaolin clay and agar agar powder. Stir well to combine.

3 Add luster dust powder or mica. You can also add biodegradable glitter or jojoba beads to add more sparkle! Stir all the ingredients until they're well combined.

4 Scoop the mixture into the airtight container. Store until you're ready to mix up a mask.

Continued on next page ▶

HOW TO USE:

1 Pour ¼ cup water into a small saucepan over high heat.

2 Once water starts to simmer, add 1 heaping teaspoon face powder. Let boil about 30 seconds while you stir the mixture. Take the saucepan off the heat and pour the mixture into a heatproof bowl. Sprinkle an extra pinch of biodegradable glitter or jojoba beads on top.

3 Let the mask cool down to room temperature and thicken at least 10 minutes. The mask should be spreadable but should have cooled down enough so that it's safe to use on your skin. Do a patch test on your arm first to check the temperature.

4 Apply a thick, even layer on a clean, dry face using clean fingers or a clean makeup brush. Let the mask sit 5–10 minutes and peel off.

5 Rinse well with water to remove any remaining traces of the mask.

HOW TO STORE:

Store in a cool, dry place and keep all water out of the container. Measure the amount you need only when you're ready to mix your mask. The face mask powder can keep up to 6 months.

JIGGLE JUICE MASK

Inspired by Dr. Jart+'s Shake & Shot Rubber Masks

This face mask is as fun to make as it is to apply on your skin!

MAKES 1 FACE MASK

$\frac{1}{2}$ cup water

$\frac{1}{4}$ teaspoon agar agar powder

Heatproof and leakproof container with a lid

1 tablespoon bentonite clay

1 tablespoon rice flour

1 tablespoon finely ground (colloidal) oatmeal

HOW TO MAKE:

1 Pour water into a small saucepan. Add agar agar powder and stir.

2 Bring the mixture to a boil. Keep stirring the mixture and let boil 1 minute.

3 Take the saucepan off the heat and allow to cool 1 minute. Pour the mixture into the container.

4 Add bentonite clay, rice flour, and oatmeal to the container.

5 Secure the lid on the container. This is a hot liquid, so make sure the lid is on tight!

6 Carefully shake the container to combine ingredients.

7 Pour the contents into a small dish or mixing bowl.

8 Let the mixture cool down to room temperature 10 minutes. It will start to thicken.

HOW TO USE:

1 Make sure the mixture has cooled down to room temperature. Do a patch test on your arm or hand first to check the temperature.

2 Use a makeup brush or your fingers to apply a thick layer on your skin. Allow the mask to sit 5–10 minutes.

3 Peel off the mask. Rinse with water.

HOW TO STORE:

This face mask is meant for a single, immediate use.

What Is Agar Agar?

Agar agar powder is made from seaweed. When you dissolve it in boiling water, it develops a jellylike consistency. It's a common ingredient in Asian desserts, and it is now becoming popular worldwide as a vegan alternative to gelatin.

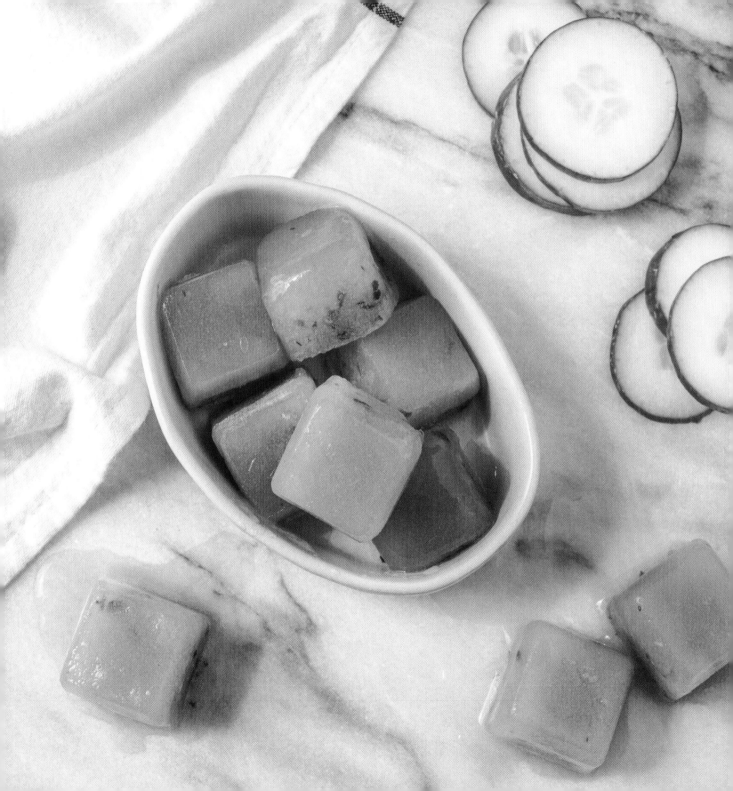

COOL AS A CUBE EYE MASK

Inspired by Yes To's Cucumbers Soothing Eye Gel

This refreshing treat will surely wake you up. The cold will de-puff any bags underneath your eyes, while the aloe vera gel and cucumber will soothe and refresh.

MAKES 3–4 ICE CUBES

½ cup water

1 tea bag pure green tea

1 (1") piece organic cucumber

¼ cup aloe vera gel

Silicone ice cube tray

HOW TO MAKE:

1 First make a cup of tea: pour water into a small saucepan and bring it to a boil. Let it boil for a few more minutes.

2 Take the saucepan off the heat and pour water into a cup. Add bag of green tea and let it steep while the tea cools down to room temperature.

3 Dice cucumber into small pieces with a kitchen knife.

4 Place cucumber pieces, aloe vera gel, and room-temperature green tea in a blender. Blend until smooth.

5 Pour the mixture into the ice cube tray. Freeze 1–2 hours until solid.

HOW TO USE:

1 Take an ice cube out of the freezer and let it sit at room temperature about 1 minute. Run it under warm water if it still feels too cold.

2 Gently massage your under-eye area. Don't use the ice cube for too long, as you could get an ice burn. Avoid getting any of the mush into your eyes.

3 Let the mixture sit on your face for a few minutes before rinsing it off. Run the rest of the ice cube over your face and scalp as well!

4 If you don't like the cold so much, put the ice cube in a washcloth. Let it melt until the washcloth is soaked. Gently run the washcloth over your face and rinse your face with water.

HOW TO STORE:

Put your cubes in an airtight container and keep in the freezer. Each ice cube is meant for a single use. Ice cubes are best used within 1 month.

LIQUID GOLD FACE MASK

Inspired by Farmacy's Honey Potion Renewing Antioxidant Hydration Mask

MAKES 1 FACE MASK

1 teaspoon organic, raw honey

Sometimes one ingredient can do all the work on its own. Honey really is worth its weight in gold. The sticky stuff has antibacterial and antioxidant properties, making it a great gentle face cleansing mask for acne-prone skin types. This mask is so gentle that you could even use it daily.

Should I Go Manuka?

Quite a few recipes in this book list honey as an ingredient. I recommend that you always use good-quality, organic, and raw honey. The benefits of New Zealand's manuka honey are established, but researchers are looking into other kinds of honey as well. As long as you use good-quality honey, you'll reap the benefits.

HOW TO MAKE:

Scoop honey out of the jar with a clean, dry spoon into a small dish or bowl.

HOW TO USE:

1 Apply a thick layer of honey on a clean face. Gently massage your face, avoiding the area around your eyes and your hairline.

2 Once you're finished with your massage, rinse it off with plenty of water. You'll be surprised how easily this sticky goo rinses from your face.

HOW TO STORE:

Store some honey for face mask purposes in a separate airtight container in a cool, dry place. Keep all water out of the container. If kept with care, this honey should have the same expiration date as the one on the original honey jar.

MIX IT UP MASKS

Inspired by Sephora Collection's Clay Mask

Clays have absorbing properties. They detoxify your skin by drawing impurities out. White kaolin clay and pink clay are great choices for sensitive skin types. Bentonite clay and Moroccan lava clay are excellent for oily and acne-prone skin types. To turn your clay into a face mask, you'll need a liquid. Add milk or yogurt if you want some gentle exfoliation, as they naturally contain lactic acid. You can also add water, flower water, or honey for extra moisture.

HOW TO MAKE:

1 Scoop clay into a small mixing bowl and add liquid of your choice.

2 Combine until the mixture turns into a paste. Add more clay or liquid until you get the desired consistency.

HOW TO USE:

1 Apply an even layer on a clean, dry face using a makeup brush or clean fingers.

2 Let the mask sit about 10 minutes. Depending on the type of liquid you use, the mask may dry faster.

3 Rinse your face with plenty of water. Follow with a mild toner or flower water to remove every bit of the mask.

HOW TO STORE:

This face mask is meant for a single, immediate use.

MAKES 1 FACE MASK

2 teaspoons of your favorite clay

1 tablespoon liquid of your choice

Now Mix It Up!

You might find it hard to determine your skin type, as it can seem like no two areas on your face are the same. Use a bentonite clay and milk mask on your forehead to absorb excess oil. Make a Moroccan lava clay and water mask to draw impurities from your nose and chin. And a pink clay and flower water mask is perfect for the sensitive area on your cheeks. Now take a look in the mirror and behold your masterpiece!

MORNING OATS FACE MASK

Inspired by St. Ives's Gentle Smoothing Oatmeal Scrub & Mask

MAKES 1 FACE MASK

1 tablespoon finely ground (colloidal) oatmeal

1 teaspoon honey

1 teaspoon plain Greek yogurt

Looking for the gentlest scrub in the universe? Look no more. Yogurt, honey, and oatmeal work together to gently exfoliate your skin.

HOW TO MAKE:

Combine oatmeal, honey, and yogurt in a small mixing bowl. Stir together until the mixture forms a paste.

HOW TO USE:

1 Apply an even layer all over your clean, dry face using a makeup brush or clean fingers. Gently massage the mask over your face with your fingertips.

2 Once you're finished with your massage, rinse with plenty of water.

HOW TO STORE:

This food-based face mask is meant for a single, immediate use.

Ground Your Oats

"Colloidal" oatmeal might sound fancy, but it just means that the oatmeal has been ground to a very fine powder consistency. You can buy this readily made in the store or you can DIY. Check the recipe for Bath Powder in Chapter 6 to make your own. Sift the oatmeal through a very fine-mesh sieve to only keep the fine particles. Or you can leave the coarser bits for a more effective scrub!

PETAL POWER MASK

Inspired by Origins' Flower Fusion Sheet Masks

This is the best-smelling face mask in this book. And it's a powerful one too. Geranium oil balances the skin, while olive oil and rose water plump and hydrate.

MAKES 1 (0.5-OUNCE) FACE MASK

0.3 ounce olive oil

1 drop geranium essential oil

0.2 ounce rose water

1 cotton sheet mask

HOW TO MAKE:

1 Pour olive oil into a small mixing bowl.

2 Add no more than 1 drop of essential oil. Stir until oils are combined.

3 Add rose water to the mixture and stir until water and oils are well combined.

4 Pour the mixture onto a clean plate and spread it out evenly. Place the sheet mask onto the plate and let it soak up the mixture.

HOW TO USE:

1 Place the mask on your clean, dry face and pat down with your fingertips.

2 Let the mask sit 5–10 minutes. Remove the mask and thoroughly rinse your face with water.

HOW TO STORE:

This sheet mask is meant for a single, immediate use.

MYSTIC MUD MASK

Inspired by Glamglow's Supermud Clearing Treatment

MAKES 0.7 OUNCE FACE MASK POWDER (ABOUT 12 APPLICATIONS)

6 tablespoons white kaolin clay

1 tablespoon activated charcoal

1 (1-ounce) airtight container

About Activated Charcoal

Not to be confused with what you'd use for a barbecue, activated charcoal is typically made from a natural source, like bamboo or coconut shells. Its absorption abilities have made it a popular at-home remedy for removing surface stains from teeth and a popular ingredient in a pore-clearing face mask.

This recipe uses the absorbing power of kaolin clay and activated charcoal to clear your pores. This face mask powder can be turned into a mask whenever it's needed.

HOW TO MAKE:

1 Combine kaolin clay and activated charcoal in a small mixing bowl. Stir well.

2 Transfer the mixture to the airtight container.

HOW TO USE:

1 When you're ready to use your mask, mix 1–2 teaspoons of the mixture with an equal amount of water. Stir until it forms a paste.

2 Apply an even layer on your face with a clean, dry makeup brush or clean fingers. Avoid your mouth and eye area. Leave on the mask 10–15 minutes.

3 Remove the face mask from your skin with a damp cloth.

HOW TO STORE:

Store face mask powder in a cool, dry place up to 6 months. Mix face mask powder with water only right before you want to use it.

SALAD FACE MASK

Inspired by Peter Thomas Roth's Cucumber Gel Mask

Make a floral salad for your face! Both cucumber and chamomile are known for their soothing effect on the skin.

MAKES 1 FACE MASK

1 (½") piece cucumber, peeled

1 tablespoon chamomile-infused sweet almond oil (see sidebar)

1 tablespoon aloe vera gel

HOW TO MAKE:

1 Dice cucumber into small pieces with a kitchen knife.

2 Add cucumber pieces, infused sweet almond oil, and aloe vera gel to a high-speed blender. Blend until you have a smooth paste.

HOW TO USE:

1 Apply an even layer on your face using a clean makeup brush or clean fingers.

2 Let the mask sit 10 minutes.

3 Rinse your face with plenty of water. Use a washcloth to remove every bit of face mask.

HOW TO STORE:

This face mask is meant for a single, immediate use.

How to Make Chamomile-Infused Sweet Almond Oil

Infuse sweet almond oil with dried chamomile flowers following the instructions at the beginning of Chapter 5. Infuse ½ cup sweet almond oil with about ¼ cup dried chamomile flowers. Keep the infused oil in an airtight container for up to 6 months. With this infused oil you can also make the Floral Soap in Chapter 3 and the Eczema Eraser Balm in Chapter 5.

WIPE OUT NOSE MASK

Inspired by Sephora Collection's Charcoal Nose Strip

MAKES 1 NOSE MASK

1 heaping teaspoon Mystic Mud Mask powder (see recipe in this chapter)

1 teaspoon plain Greek or full-fat yogurt

Here's a mask to wipe out those stubborn blackheads on your nose. The lactic acid from the yogurt will gently exfoliate, while the Mystic Mud Mask will draw out your skin's impurities.

HOW TO MAKE:

In a small mixing bowl combine Mystic Mud Mask powder and yogurt until the ingredients form a paste.

HOW TO USE:

1 Apply a thick layer of the paste across your nose. You can use any leftovers on the rest of your T-zone, like your forehead or chin.

2 Let the mask dry 5–10 minutes and then rinse it off.

3 Use a damp cloth or a cotton pad with a mild toner or flower water to remove any remaining traces of the mask.

HOW TO STORE:

This nose mask is meant for a single, immediate use.

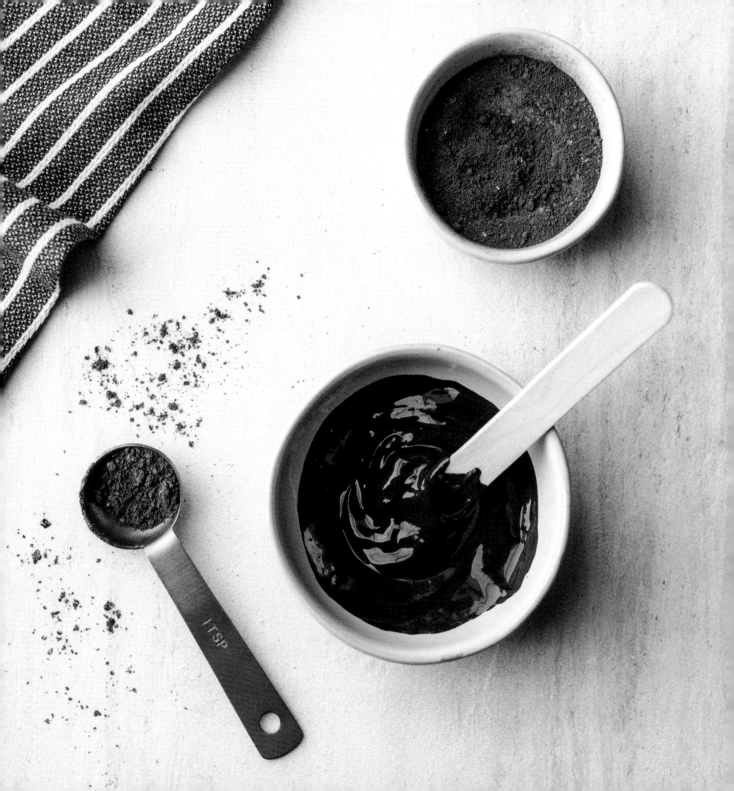

STRAWBERRY SHAKE MASK

Inspired by Mario Badescu's Strawberry Face Scrub

MAKES 1 FACE MASK

1 organic strawberry

1 tablespoon plain Greek yogurt

1 tablespoon honey

This mild exfoliating face mask uses strawberries, a natural source of vitamin C.

HOW TO MAKE:

1 Dice strawberry and put the pieces into a small mixing bowl. Mush with a fork until strawberry turns into a paste.

2 Add yogurt and honey to the mixing bowl.

3 Stir with a spoon or fork until all the ingredients are combined.

HOW TO USE:

1 Apply an even layer all over your clean face using a clean makeup brush or clean fingers. Gently massage your face with your fingertips.

2 Let the mask sit 10 minutes, then rinse your face with water.

HOW TO STORE:

This food-based face mask is meant for a single, immediate use.

SUDS MASK

Inspired by Sephora Collection's Supermask—The Bubble Mask

This mask starts to foam when you touch it! You can swap the fractionated coconut oil in this mask for another carrier oil of your choice.

MAKES 1 FACE MASK

1 tablespoon water

1 drop unscented liquid Castile soap

1 tablespoon fractionated coconut oil

1 cotton sheet mask

HOW TO MAKE:

1 Add water and Castile soap to a small mixing bowl. Stir to dissolve the soap in the water.

2 Add coconut oil. Whisk vigorously to break up coconut oil bubbles as much as possible.

3 Pour the mixture onto a large plate and spread it out evenly. Place the cotton sheet mask on top and let it soak up the mixture.

HOW TO USE:

1 Apply the sheet mask on your face and pat it down with your fingertips. Once the face mask is in place, gently massage the mask with your fingertips. The mask will start to foam.

2 Once you're finished with your massage, remove the mask and rinse your face with plenty of water.

HOW TO STORE:

This sheet mask is meant for a single, immediate use.

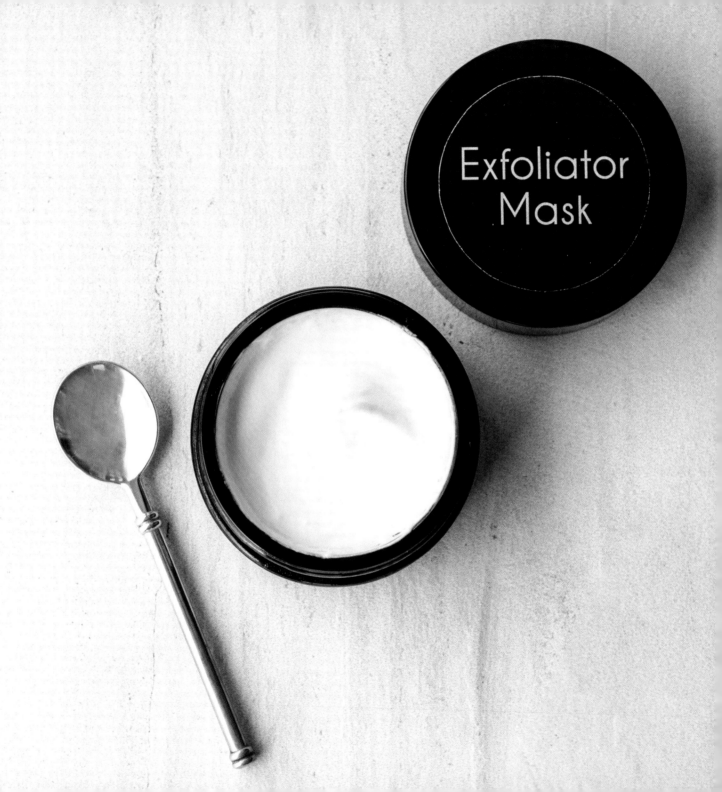

EXFOLIATOR MASK

Inspired by Dr. Brandt's Microdermabrasion Age Defying Exfoliator

The small salt crystals in this mask will scrub your face. The lactic acid in the yogurt will double the exfoliation, and the jojoba oil will soothe and balance.

MAKES 1 FACE MASK

1 teaspoon fine sea salt

1 tablespoon full-fat plain yogurt

1 teaspoon jojoba oil

HOW TO MAKE:

1 Combine sea salt, yogurt, and jojoba oil in a small mixing bowl.

2 Mix together with a spoon until the ingredients form a paste.

HOW TO USE:

1 Apply a thin layer of the paste on your clean face. Gently massage your face with your fingertips.

2 Rinse well to reveal freshly scrubbed skin. I recommend that you don't use this powerful face mask more than once a week.

HOW TO STORE:

This face mask is meant for a single, immediate use.

TEA PARTY EYE MASK

Inspired by Sephora Collection's Green Tea Eye Mask

MAKES 2 UNDER-EYE PADS

¼ cup water

1 tea bag pure green tea

1 round cotton pad

Sometimes you just have to fake having gotten a good, long beauty sleep. This easy-to-make eye mask uses the simple power of green tea to freshen your look.

HOW TO MAKE:

1 Let's start with the tea: bring water to a boil in a small saucepan.

2 Pour hot water into a cup and let cool down slightly before adding tea bag. Let tea steep while water cools down.

3 Cut cotton pad in half.

4 Once water has cooled down to room temperature, remove tea bag and pour steeped tea onto a plate.

5 Drop the cotton pad halves into the liquid and put the plate in the refrigerator for about 10 minutes.

HOW TO USE:

1 Before using your eye pads, squeeze them softly between your fingers to rinse out any excess liquid.

2 Place one pad underneath each eye. Pat them down gently with your fingertips so they won't fall off.

3 Let pads sit at least 10 minutes before taking them off.

4 Rinse your face with water and pat dry with a towel.

HOW TO STORE:

These under-eye pads are meant for a single, immediate use.

TOMATO TONER FACE WIPES

Inspired by Yes To's Tomatoes Blemish Clearing Facial Towelettes

These face wipes use the power of tomatoes. Tomato juice naturally contains alpha hydroxy acids (AHAs) that effectively remove dead skin cells.

MAKES 3–4 FACE WIPES

½ medium organic tomato, peeled

1 tablespoon witch hazel

1 tablespoon aloe vera gel

3–4 cotton pads

HOW TO MAKE:

1 Dice tomato into small chunks with a kitchen knife.

2 Add tomato, witch hazel, and aloe vera gel to a high-speed blender. Blend until smooth.

3 Distribute cotton pads on a clean plate or flat surface. Pour the mixture over the cotton pads. Give the pads a few minutes to soak up the mixture.

HOW TO USE:

1 Squeeze any excess liquid out of the cotton pads. Gently rub the cotton pads on a clean face, staying away from your eye area.

2 Thoroughly rinse your face with water. Use a damp washcloth to remove every bit of the mixture.

3 Follow with your go-to face moisturizer.

HOW TO STORE:

These face wipes are meant for immediate use. The recipe makes enough to share with one or two friends.

YOU'RE GOLDEN EYE MASK

Inspired by Peter Thomas Roth's 24K Gold Pure Luxury Lift & Firm Hydra-Gel Eye Patches

MAKES 6 EYE PATCH STRIPS

1/4 cup water

1/2 teaspoon agar agar powder

1 teaspoon raw honey

1 tablespoon coffee-infused grapeseed oil (see sidebar)

1 deep-dish plate

How to Make Coffee-Infused Grapeseed Oil

To make your own coffee-infused oil: Infuse 1/2 cup grapeseed oil with 1/4 cup dry ground coffee beans using the cold infusion method described at the beginning of Chapter 5. Store the coffee-infused oil in an airtight container up to 3 months. With this oil you can make plenty of You're Golden Eye Mask patches, or use it to make the Natural Tan Lotion in Chapter 5.

The honey and agar agar form a protective layer on the skin, while the caffeine wakes up the bags under your eyes.

HOW TO MAKE:

1 Bring water to a boil in a small saucepan. Put the lid on and let water boil at least 5 minutes.

2 Remove the lid and add agar agar powder. Stir until powder has dissolved. Let it boil for another 30 seconds.

3 Take the saucepan off the heat. Add honey and whisk until dissolved.

4 Add coffee-infused oil and whisk vigorously. Oil and water won't mix, but if you stir the mixture well, the oil will temporarily disperse in the water.

5 Pour the mixture onto the deep-dish plate. Let it set 20 minutes or until it's a firm jelly.

6 Flip the deep-dish plate onto a flat plate or cutting board and let the jelly fall out.

7 Cut the jelly into 6 (1/2") strips.

HOW TO USE:

1 Place one strip underneath each eye. Pat it down with your fingertips. If the strips are thin enough, they should stay put.

2 Leave strips on about 10 minutes.

3 Remove strips and wipe away any oils with a damp cloth.

HOW TO STORE:

Each strip is meant for a single use. Store unused eye strips in an airtight container in the refrigerator for no more than 3 days.

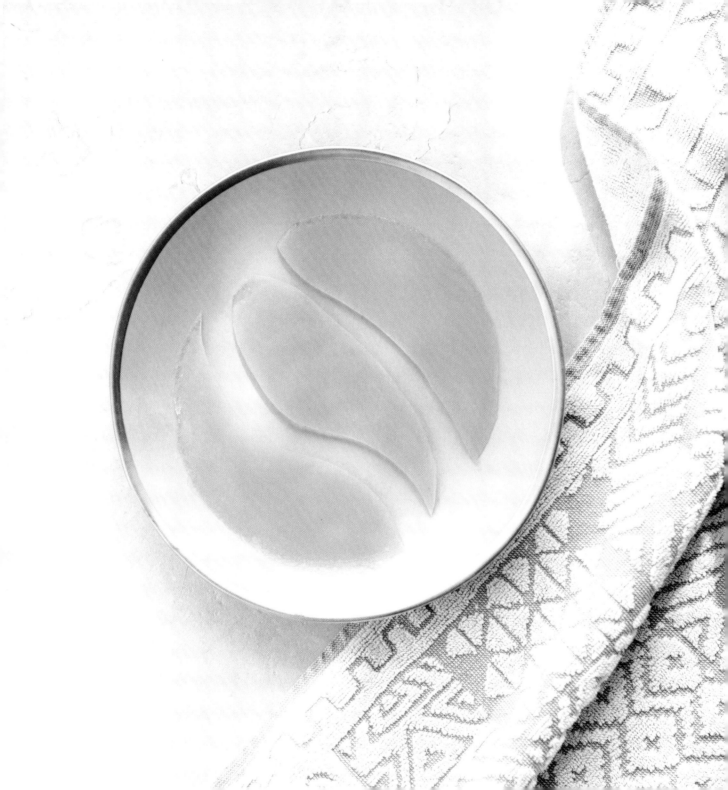

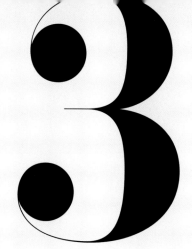

CHAPTER 3
SHINE THERAPY

I've learned the hard way that when it comes to your beauty routine, less really is more. I watched bloggers and YouTubers use one product after the other, and I thought I needed to do the same to find the perfect skincare products for me.

After a while my skin got tired of constantly adjusting to new products, and it started to show it. My skin was always either oily or dry. So I tried other products to fix the problem. You see where I'm going with this? Now I keep my beauty routine easy and simple. For a moisturizer, I've switched to a simple face oil. (You can find my favorite skincare oils in this chapter.) I even stopped using conditioner and swapped it for a weekly moisturizing hair mask.

In this chapter you'll find my favorite skincare basics to give your skin and hair some much-needed shine therapy. Mix and match your favorite products and make them part of your personal natural beauty routine. It's time to bring back that shine!

Carrier Oils Nourish Your Skin

Your mind might go straight to cooking when you think of oils, but your skin finds them just as delicious! Oils made from nuts, seeds, or plants have wonderful benefits for your skin. Look for cold-pressed oils or extra-virgin oils, as they are generally preferred over refined oils. Unrefined oils maintain more of the essential nutrients your skin loves so much.

Let's take a closer look at some of the oils used in the recipes in this book:

- **Castor oil:** Castor oil is a heavy oil, and the skin absorbs it very slowly. That's why you use it in combination with another carrier oil for a face or body oil. It leaves a nice protective layer on your skin. It also has a glossy finish, which is why I like to use it in lip balms, serums, lip glosses, and cream eye shadows.

- **Coconut oil:** Unlike other plant-based oils, cold-pressed coconut oil is solid at room temperature. This powerful oil also has antibacterial and antiviral properties, making it a winner for DIY beauty products.

- **Grapeseed oil:** This is my personal favorite because the skin absorbs this oil pretty quickly, and it doesn't leave a greasy film behind. This oil is also praised for its antibacterial and anti-inflammatory properties.

- **Jojoba oil:** Jojoba oil is actually a liquid wax. This oil has the amazing ability to form a thin layer on the surface of your skin to protect it. Your skin can still breathe naturally, but at the same time the jojoba oil keeps the skin smooth, soft, and moisturized.

- **Sweet almond oil:** This is a top pick for dry skin types, as it is high in vitamin D. We'll use this versatile oil in bath bombs, body balms, and even soaps.

- **Vitamin E oil:** This oil gets a special mention because vitamin E is considered an antioxidant. It helps keep the other oils in your recipe from going bad. As soon as a plant-based oil comes into contact with air or light, it will start to oxidize. This natural process causes your oil to go rancid after a while. You can slow down this process by adding an antioxidant. A little vitamin E goes a long way. Typically, 1 percent is enough to prolong the shelf life of your oils. I like to add a few drops of vitamin E oil when I'm using oils with a shorter shelf life, like grapeseed oil and evening primrose oil.

Vitamin E is not a preservative! You will still need to keep all contaminants out of your homemade products. See Chapter 1 to learn more about how to keep your homemade products safe.

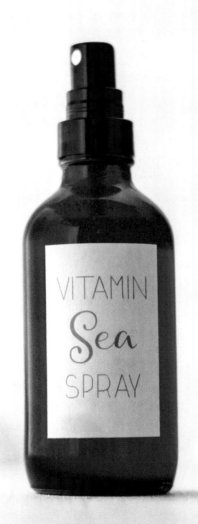

VITAMIN SEA SPRAY

Inspired by Bumble and bumble's Surf Spray

Rock those beachy waves all year round. The salt will encourage your hair to curl, the aloe vera gel will help hold the curls, and the oils will moisturize your locks.

MAKES 1 (4.3-OUNCE) SPRAY

½ cup water

1 teaspoon sea salt

1 teaspoon aloe vera gel

1 teaspoon fractionated coconut oil

3 drops lavender essential oil

1 (4.5-ounce) spray bottle

HOW TO MAKE:

1 Bring water to a boil in a small saucepan. Put the lid on and let water boil at least 5 minutes. Remove the lid and take the saucepan off the heat.

2 Add sea salt and aloe vera gel to water and mix with a whisk until salt and aloe vera gel have dissolved. Set aside and let the mixture cool to room temperature.

3 Pour coconut oil into a small mixing bowl. Add lavender essential oil and stir to combine.

4 Add the cooled water mixture to the mixing bowl. Whisk to combine the ingredients.

5 Use a small funnel to pour the mixture into the spray bottle. Screw on the nozzle and it's ready for use!

HOW TO USE:

1 The water and oils in this recipe won't mix on their own, as we're not using an emulsifier. So give the bottle a good shake before each use.

2 Spray liberally on dry or damp hair. Scrunch your hair upward using your hands to encourage your strands to make waves.

3 Leave a few minutes to dry.

HOW TO STORE:

This is a water-based product. Store in the refrigerator and use within 3–5 days.

ARGAN HAIR OIL

Inspired by Moroccanoil's Moroccanoil Treatment

MAKES 1 (0.7-OUNCE) HAIR SERUM

0.5 ounce argan oil

0.2 ounce flaxseed oil

1 (1-ounce) dropper bottle

Argan and flaxseed oil are super oils for your hair. Use this combo to bring shine to frayed ends.

HOW TO MAKE:

Using a small funnel or pipet, transfer argan oil and flaxseed oil into the clean, dry dropper bottle.

HOW TO USE:

1 Put a drop of hair oil in the palm of your hand. Rub your hands together to spread the oil evenly.

2 Run your fingers and palms through your hair to coat the ends. Style your hair like you normally would.

HOW TO STORE:

Store this hair oil in the refrigerator up to 1 month.

AVO EYE CREAM

Inspired by Kiehl's Creamy Eye Treatment with Avocado

The ingredient combo in this eye cream is perfect to moisturize the fragile skin around your eyes, leaving your under-eye area looking fresh and relaxed!

MAKES 1 (0.5-OUNCE) EYE CREAM

1 tablespoon shea butter

1 tablespoon avocado oil

1 (0.5-ounce) airtight container

HOW TO MAKE:

1 Slowly melt shea butter in a double boiler over medium heat. Or melt shea butter in a heatproof container in the microwave on a low setting (650 watts or lower) using 1-minute intervals. Stir between intervals until shea butter has melted.

2 Take the double boiler off the heat or take the container out of the microwave. Add avocado oil to melted shea butter and stir to combine.

3 Let the mixture solidify 1–2 hours at room temperature or place covered in the refrigerator to speed up the cooling process.

4 Once solid, mix lightly with a fork or whisk to create a creamy texture. Scoop the eye cream into the airtight container.

HOW TO USE:

1 Each night before you go to bed dab a tiny amount of eye cream underneath your eyes. Don't apply it directly underneath your lower eyelashes. Apply it about ½" away from your eyes instead, as eye creams tend to move upward as you sleep.

2 Wake up the next day looking completely refreshed.

HOW TO STORE:

Store in a cool, dry place out of direct sunlight up to 6 months.

BEAUTY SLEEP SPRAY

Inspired by Earth Therapeutics' Elixir of Dreams Pillow Mist

MAKES 1 (2-OUNCE) SPRAY

1 (2.5-ounce) spray bottle

1.5 ounces witch hazel

0.5 ounce high-proof (at least 90 percent) alcohol

20 drops lavender essential oil

Need help catching some sleep? A few spritzes of this lavender-scented sleep spray will have you dreaming in no time.

HOW TO MAKE:

1 Unscrew the dispenser top from the spray bottle and insert a small funnel.

2 Carefully pour witch hazel and alcohol into the bottle.

3 Take the funnel out of the bottle and add essential oil.

4 Screw the top back on tightly and shake until all the ingredients are combined.

HOW TO USE:

1 Shake the bottle before each use.

2 Spray this mist a few times on your pillow and bed sheets. Give the spray a few seconds to evaporate. Don't spray directly into your face. And be careful when you spray around pets and small children.

HOW TO STORE:

The alcohol acts as a preservative, so this sleep spray should keep up to 6 months.

CLEAN WIPES

Inspired by Pacifica's Underarm Deodorant Wipes

With one quick swipe you leave a layer of antibacterial coconut oil, good-smelling essential oils, and absorbing clay behind.

HOW TO MAKE:

1 Melt coconut oil in a double boiler over medium heat. Or melt coconut oil in a heatproof container in the microwave on a low setting (650 watts or lower) for 1 minute or until coconut oil has melted.

2 Take the double boiler off the heat or take the heatproof container out of the microwave. Add arrowroot powder and kaolin clay to the melted oil and stir well to combine the ingredients. Set aside.

3 Distribute cotton pads evenly on a clean plate.

4 Add essential oils to the melted mixture and stir to evenly distribute the oils.

5 Use a spoon to drizzle about 1 teaspoon of the mixture onto each pad.

6 Place the pads covered in the refrigerator for 1–2 hours and let them soak up the mixture.

7 Once the mixture has turned solid, you can stack the cotton pads and store them in an airtight container.

HOW TO USE:

1 Make sure your skin is clean and dry before using. Take a cotton pad out of the container and swipe it on both armpits.

MAKES 2.5 OUNCES OF DEODORANT (ABOUT 20 COTTON PADS)

2 ounces coconut oil

1 tablespoon arrowroot powder

1 tablespoon kaolin clay

20 round cotton pads

5–10 drops essential oils of your choice

2 Give your skin a few minutes to soak up the oil. Use a new cotton pad each time.

HOW TO STORE:

If you live in a warm climate (or if temperatures are high), the coconut oil might melt. Keep these wipes in the refrigerator if you want to keep the coconut oil solid. You can keep these wipes in an airtight container up to 6 months.

COCONDITIONER

Inspired by Not Your Mother's Naturals' Coconut Milk & African Marula Tree Oil High Moisture Conditioner

MAKES 1 HAIR MASK FOR MEDIUM–LONG HAIR

½ cup canned full-fat coconut milk

1 tablespoon extra-virgin olive oil

This exotic hair mask uses creamy coconut to smooth frayed hair. Use instead of your conditioner for shiny locks!

HOW TO MAKE:

1 Set can of coconut milk in the refrigerator at least 24 hours before making this recipe.

2 Scoop the creamy top layer out of the can into a medium mixing bowl.

3 Add olive oil. Stir with a spoon until the ingredients are blended.

HOW TO USE:

1 Slather the mask on your hair, focusing on the ends. Cover your hair with a shower cap or twist it up into a bun.

2 Let the mask sit 10–30 minutes and then rinse it out. You might want to shampoo twice to get all of the mask out.

HOW TO STORE:

This food-based hair mask is meant for a single, immediate use.

'NANAS HAIR MASK

Inspired by The Body Shop's Banana Truly Nourishing Conditioner

Let's go bananas on our hair. This hair mask is like an energy smoothie for your strands!

MAKES 1 HAIR MASK

½ medium ripe banana

1 tablespoon plain full-fat yogurt

1 tablespoon coconut oil

HOW TO MAKE:

1 Add banana, yogurt, and coconut oil to a high-speed blender. Blend the ingredients until they form a paste.

2 Use a sieve to make sure you are left with a smooth paste (any remaining banana chunks will stick to your hair like crazy).

HOW TO USE:

1 Slather the mixture on your hair, from the roots to the ends. Cover your hair with a shower cap or twist it up into a bun.

2 Let the mixture sit about 10 minutes.

3 Rinse the mask out thoroughly before washing your hair like you normally would. You might want to shampoo twice to get all of the mask out.

HOW TO STORE:

This food-based hair mask is meant for a single, immediate use.

BLUSH FACE SPRAY

Inspired by Herbivore Botanicals' Rose Hibiscus Coconut Water Hydrating Face Mist

MAKES 1 (2-OUNCE) FACE SPRAY

1 cup water

1 tea bag pure hibiscus tea

1 (2-ounce) spray bottle

1 ounce rose water

About Flower Waters

Good-quality flower waters (also called hydrosols) are natural by-products from making essential oils. The most common ones are rose water and witch hazel, but you can also find other hydrosols like lavender, tea tree, and orange blossom flower water. Check the ingredient list before you buy a flower water. Some flower waters sold in stores are just water mixed with essential oils and other additives, and they can smell very artificial.

Nothing beats a floral-scented refreshing spray on a hot summer day!

HOW TO MAKE:

1 Pour water into a small saucepan and put the lid on. Bring water to a boil and let it boil 5 minutes.

2 Take the saucepan off the heat and carefully pour water into a cup. Add tea bag to the cup and let it steep while water cools down to room temperature.

3 Unscrew the top of the spray bottle and pour rose water into the bottle. Fill the rest of the bottle with the cooled hibiscus tea.

4 Screw the top back on and it's ready for use.

HOW TO USE:

Since this spray is stored in the refrigerator, the cooled mixture will be extra refreshing! Take the spray out of the refrigerator and mist your face, arms, and/or legs liberally. Repeat as many times as needed.

HOW TO STORE:

Store this face spray in the refrigerator and use within 1 day.

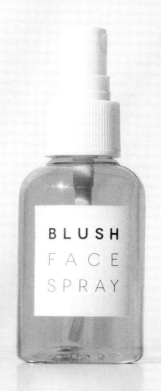

NO 'POO POWDER

Inspired by Bumble and bumble's Brownish Hair Powder

MAKES ABOUT 1.5 OUNCES OF DRY SHAMPOO POWDER

3 tablespoons rice flour

3 tablespoons arrowroot powder

1 tablespoon white kaolin clay

1–3 tablespoons cocoa powder

1 (2-ounce) airtight container

This DIY dry shampoo powder doesn't leave a greasy film like some dry shampoos. And we snuck in some antioxidant-rich cocoa powder that'll save you from embarrassing white residue.

HOW TO MAKE:

1 Combine rice flour, arrowroot powder, and kaolin clay in a medium mixing bowl and stir well.

2 Add 1–3 tablespoons cocoa powder depending on the color of your hair. Stir until the mixture has an even color.

3 Scoop the mixture into the airtight container.

HOW TO USE:

1 Sprinkle a little bit of powder on your roots. Massage your hair with your fingertips to work the powder into your hair.

2 Brush out any residue.

HOW TO STORE:

Store in a cool, dry place and keep all water out of the container. This dry shampoo powder can keep up to 6 months.

PASSION FOR OIL

Inspired by Tarte's Maracuja Oil

Maracuja oil is simply an oil made from the seeds of passion fruits. It's a lightweight oil rich in antioxidants. Use this alone as a face oil or over your favorite moisturizer as a face serum. You can also use this oil on dry cuticles, on rough patches, or as a hair serum.

MAKES 1 (1-OUNCE) FACE SERUM

1 ounce passion fruit seed oil

1 (1.5-ounce) dark amber dropper bottle

HOW TO MAKE:

Use a small funnel to pour passion fruit seed oil into the dropper bottle.

HOW TO USE:

1 Place a few drops in the palm of your hand. Rub your hands together to lightly heat up the oil.

2 Apply on your face and massage it in with your fingertips.

HOW TO STORE:

Passion fruit seed oil can have a shelf life of 1–2 years. Check the expiration date on the original packaging. Don't forget to label your dropper bottle.

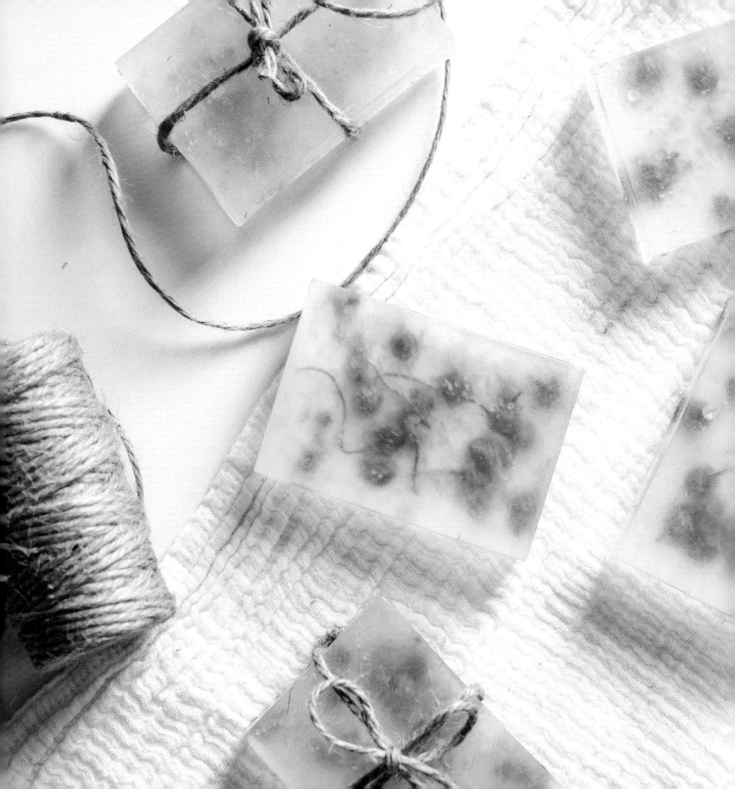

FLORAL SOAP

Inspired by Korres's Chamomile Softening Soap

If you're looking for a gentle soap option, this would be the go-to choice for sensitive skin types. Plant-based glycerin and chamomile-infused sweet almond oil soothe your skin.

HOW TO MAKE:

1 Dice glycerin soap into ½" cubes. Place the cubes in a heatproof container and melt in the microwave on a low setting (650 watts or lower) using 30-second intervals. Check between each interval to see if the soap has melted. You can also use the double boiler method to melt the soap pieces.

2 Add chamomile-infused sweet almond oil to the melted soap. Stir to combine.

3 Pour the soap mixture into the mold. If you want, you can scatter dried chamomile flowers over the wet soap. Let sit at room temperature 1–2 hours or until it has cooled and is hard.

HOW TO USE:

Run this soap over wet skin. Rinse with water.

HOW TO STORE:

Let the soap bar air-dry after each use. To give it as a gift, wrap it in craft wrapping paper once it is cooled and hard. This soap can keep up to 6 months.

MAKES 1 (4.5-OUNCE) SOAP BAR

4 ounces unscented, pure glycerin soap

2 tablespoons chamomile-infused sweet almond oil (see sidebar)

1 rectangular or square soap mold

1 teaspoon dried chamomile flowers (optional)

How to Make Chamomile-Infused Sweet Almond Oil

To make your own chamomile-infused sweet almond oil, try this: Infuse ½ cup of sweet almond oil with about ¼ cup of dried chamomile flowers. Choose either the hot or cold infusion method and follow the instructions at the beginning of Chapter 5. Keep the chamomile-infused oil in an airtight container up to 6 months. With this infused oil you can also make the Salad Face Mask in Chapter 2 and the Eczema Eraser Balm in Chapter 5.

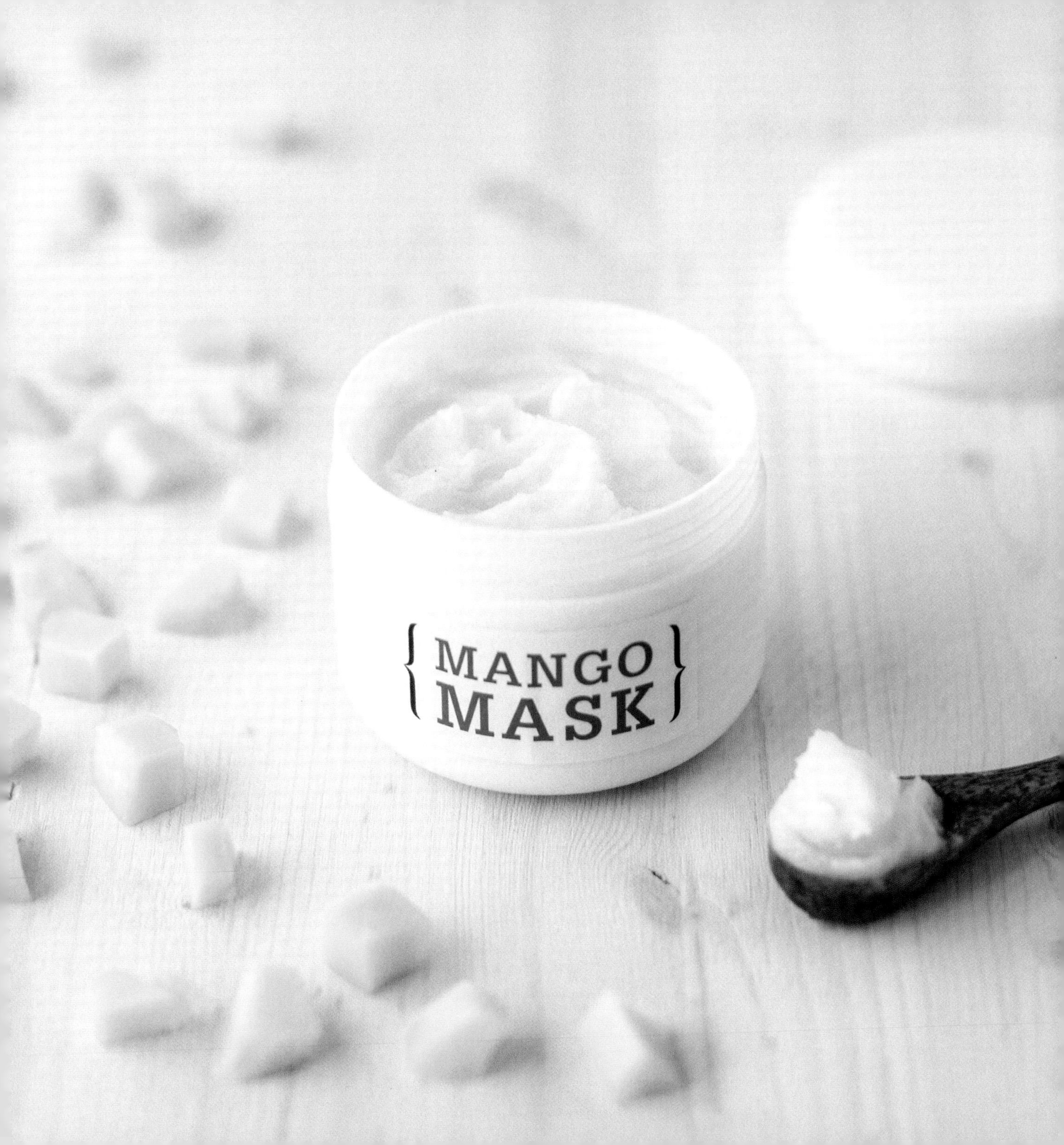
{MANGO
MASK}

MANGO MASK

Inspired by Not Your Mother's Beach Babe Butter Masque

This hair mask might just be the solution those of you with very dry hair or split ends have been waiting for.

MAKES 1 (3-OUNCE) HAIR MASK

0.7 ounce mango butter

1.5 ounces coconut oil

0.8 ounce grapeseed oil

1 (3.5-ounce) airtight container

HOW TO MAKE:

1 Melt mango butter in a double boiler over medium heat. Or place in a heatproof container and melt in the microwave on a low setting (650 watts or lower) using 1-minute intervals until the butter has melted.

2 Take the double boiler off the heat or take the container out of the microwave. Add coconut oil and stir until it has dissolved.

3 Add grapeseed oil and stir until all ingredients are combined, then pour into the airtight container. Give the mask 3–5 hours to set before you use it.

HOW TO USE:

1 Scoop 1–2 teaspoons out of the container depending on the length of your hair. Rub the mask on your hair, focusing on the ends. Avoid the scalp and roots.

2 Comb the mask through your hair with a wide-tooth comb until your hair is evenly coated. Let it sit 10–30 minutes.

3 Shampoo as you normally would. Shampoo twice if necessary to get all of the mask out.

4 You can also use this mask as a leave-in conditioner! Scoop out a pea-sized amount and rub it between your hands. Run your fingers through wet hair, focusing on the ends.

HOW TO STORE:

Store in a cool, dark place and keep all water out of the container. This hair mask can keep up to 6 months.

PINK PETAL FACE SERUM

Inspired by Korres's Wild Rose Advanced Brightening & Nourishing Face Oil

Rosehip oil is naturally infused with rose petals in this pretty-looking face serum. This lightweight oil is used to treat acne, wrinkles, dark under-eye circles, and scars. Use this on its own as a facial oil or on top of your moisturizer as a face serum.

MAKES 1 (2-OUNCE) FACE SERUM

1 (2.5-ounce) dropper bottle

2 ounces rosehip seed oil

10 drops vitamin E oil

3 drops rose geranium essential oil (optional)

1 teaspoon dried organic rose petals

HOW TO MAKE:

1 Insert a small funnel into the dropper bottle.

2 Carefully pour rosehip seed oil into the bottle. Remove the funnel and add vitamin E oil and essential oil, if using.

3 Add dried rose petals to the bottle. You might need to crunch them a little bit to fit them through the opening.

4 Screw the dropper cap onto the bottle. Shake the bottle vigorously to mix all the ingredients.

HOW TO USE:

1 Apply a drop or two to the palm of your hand. Lightly rub your hands together.

2 Spread the oil on your face using the palms of your hands and massage it in using your fingertips.

HOW TO STORE:

Store in a cool, dry place out of direct sunlight up to 6 weeks.

SOOTHE MY SCALP SERUM

Inspired by Philip Kingsley's Exfoliating Scalp Mask

Three essential oils work together to strengthen your hair and improve the health of your scalp.

HOW TO MAKE:

1 Combine jojoba oil and essential oils in a small mixing bowl.

2 Add aloe vera gel and stir well until all the ingredients are combined.

HOW TO USE:

1 Divide your hair into parts and massage the serum into your scalp.

2 Comb the serum through your hair with a fine-tooth comb. Let sit 5–10 minutes.

3 Rinse well and then wash your hair as you normally would.

HOW TO STORE:

This hair mask is meant for a single, immediate use.

MAKES 1 (1-OUNCE) HAIR SERUM

0.2 ounce jojoba oil

1 drop lavender essential oil

1 drop cedarwood essential oil

1 drop clary sage essential oil

0.8 ounce aloe vera gel

PROTEIN-PACKED HAIR MASK

Inspired by Moroccanoil's Restorative Hair Mask

MAKES 1 MASK FOR MEDIUM-LONG HAIR

1 small egg

1 tablespoon argan oil

3 tablespoons plain Greek yogurt

Don't forget your protein! Your hair loves it just as much as the rest of your body. This homemade mask may not match its inspired product in color because it is made with fresh, natural ingredients.

HOW TO MAKE:

1 Break egg into a small mixing bowl. Whisk yolk and egg white until combined.

2 Add argan oil and Greek yogurt. Stir until the ingredients are combined.

HOW TO USE:

1 Slather the mixture on your hair. Cover with a shower cap or twist your hair up into a bun.

2 Let the mask sit about 10 minutes before rinsing it out. Shampoo twice if necessary to get all of the mask out.

HOW TO STORE:

This hair mask is meant for a single, immediate use.

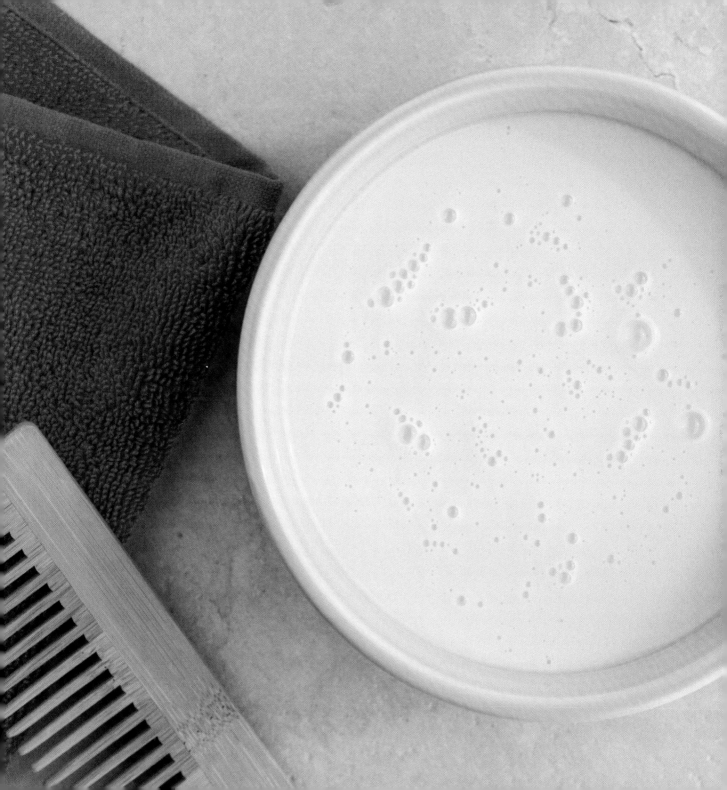

SOOTHE MY SCALP RINSE

Inspired by Philip Kingsley's Flaky Scalp Toner

MAKES 1 HAIR RINSE

1 tablespoon apple cider vinegar

3 tablespoons water

1 tablespoon olive oil

This pungent hair rinse packs a punch! The apple cider vinegar tones your scalp, and the olive oil moisturizes dry, flaky skin. But leave out the oil if you have very oily roots.

HOW TO MAKE:

Combine apple cider vinegar, water, and olive oil in a medium mixing bowl. Stir the ingredients together until olive oil is dispersed in the mixture.

HOW TO USE:

1 Flip your hair over the sink, shower, or bathtub. Pour the mixture over your hair, focusing on your scalp. Gently massage your scalp with the mixture.

2 Flip your hair back and let the mixture sit about 10 minutes.

3 Wash your hair as you normally would. Use this rinse up to once a week.

HOW TO STORE:

This food-based rinse is meant for a single, immediate use.

SCENTED BALM

Inspired by L'Occitane's Solid Perfumes

We're bringing solid oil perfumes back! Make yours unique by adding dried flowers, like rose petals, or a pinch of biodegradable glitter to your balm. For a floral-scented balm, for example, use 8 drops of rose geranium, 6 drops of lavender, and 3 drops of ylang-ylang essential oil.

MAKES 3 (0.4-OUNCE) BALMS

0.4 ounce beeswax pellets

0.8 ounce coconut oil

10–20 drops essential oil(s) of your choice

3 (0.4-ounce) airtight containers

HOW TO MAKE:

1 Slowly melt beeswax in a double boiler over medium heat.

2 Add coconut oil to beeswax and melt slowly until the mixture is liquid. Take the double boiler off the heat.

3 Add 10–20 drops essential oil(s) depending on how strong you want the finished product to smell or how sensitive your skin is to essential oils. Stir with a spoon to distribute the scent evenly.

4 Pour the mixture into the containers. Let the mixture solidify 2–3 hours before use.

HOW TO USE:

Swirl a clean, dry finger on top of the balm until you've picked up enough of the scent. Rub it on your neck and wrists.

HOW TO STORE:

Store out of direct sunlight up to 6 months. Don't forget to label the container so you don't accidently mistake your Scented Balm for a lip balm. Talk about essential oil overload!

Twist It Up!

For easy touch-ups throughout the day pour the scented balm mixture into clean, empty twist-up lip balm containers. Perfect for your handbag!

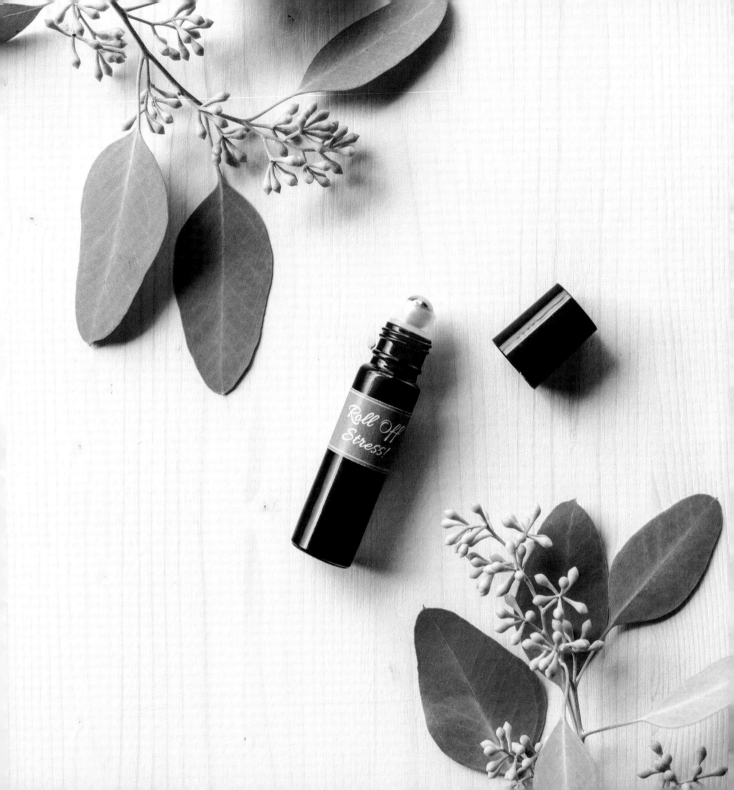

ROLL OFF STRESS!

Inspired by Bath & Body Works' Stress Relief—Eucalyptus + Spearmint Essential Oil Rollerball

Stress relief is just a whiff away. You won't be able to resist smelling your wrists after you've applied this therapy oil. If you have sensitive skin, use the smaller amounts of essential oils.

MAKES 2 (0.5-OUNCE) THERAPY OILS

1 ounce jojoba oil

1–2 drops eucalyptus essential oil

1–2 drops spearmint essential oil

2 (0.6-ounce) roller bottles

HOW TO MAKE:

1 Place jojoba oil in a small mixing bowl.

2 Add eucalyptus and spearmint essential oils. Stir well to blend all the oils.

3 Remove the caps and applicators from the roller bottles. Using a small funnel, pour the oil mixture into the bottles. Stop about ½" below the rim so the bottle won't overflow when you put the applicator back in.

HOW TO USE:

When you're in need of stress relief, apply some therapy oil on the insides of your wrists. Bring your nose close to your wrist and take a nice deep breath in.

HOW TO STORE:

Store in a cool, dry place out of direct sunlight up to 6 months.

Try Another Scent!

If eucalyptus or spearmint isn't one of your favorite scents, you can experiment with another calming essential oil, like lavender or sandalwood.

SQUEAKY GREEN DEODORANT

Inspired by Tarte's Clean Queen Vegan Deodorant

MAKES 1 (1.6-OUNCE) DEODORANT

0.9 ounce cocoa butter

0.2 ounce coconut oil

1 tablespoon bentonite clay

1 tablespoon arrowroot powder

1/2 tablespoon baking soda

6 drops essential oil of your choice

1 (2-ounce) twist-up container

Choose Your Scent

The great thing about making your own deodorant is that you can choose your own scent. Patchouli is a popular choice, as its earthy scent lingers for a long time. It pairs great with geranium, lavender, or vanilla. As the skin underneath your arms is very sensitive, it's best to avoid strong essential oils, like peppermint and lemongrass.

It's green and keeps you smelling squeaky clean! If you have very sensitive skin, leave out the baking soda and let the clay, arrowroot powder, and essential oil prevent you from getting sweaty, smelly armpits.

HOW TO MAKE:

1 Melt cocoa butter in a double boiler over medium heat.

2 Add coconut oil and stir to combine.

3 Take the double boiler off the heat and stir in bentonite clay, arrowroot powder, and baking soda.

4 Add essential oil and stir well to make sure it is spread evenly throughout the mixture.

5 Make sure the twist-up mechanism of your container is wound all the way down to the bottom. Pour the melted mixture into the container.

6 Give the deodorant about 2–3 hours to set before using. Place it covered in the refrigerator to speed up the cooling process.

HOW TO USE:

Apply a thin layer on clean, dry skin. One swipe is all it takes! Give the deodorant a few minutes to dry before getting dressed.

HOW TO STORE:

Store in a cool, dry place out of direct sunlight up to 6 months.

THE DAILY SCRUB

Inspired by Dermalogica's Daily Microfoliant

This scrub is so gentle that you can use it on repeat. Use this face scrub according to your own preference. I like to use this scrub every 2 to 3 days.

HOW TO MAKE:

1 Place white tea leaves in a shallow bowl or on a small plate. Crush leaves with the back of a spoon until you have a fine powder. Remove any hard bits, like stems and twigs.

2 In a medium mixing bowl combine colloidal oatmeal, rice flour, and crushed tea leaves. Stir with a spoon to combine the ingredients.

3 Transfer powder to the airtight container.

HOW TO USE:

1 Scoop about 1 teaspoon of powder into the palm of your hand or into a mixing bowl. Add 1 teaspoon water and mix into a paste.

2 Apply the paste on your clean face and massage with your fingertips.

3 Rinse with plenty of water. Follow with a mild toner or flower water to remove all bits of the paste.

HOW TO STORE:

Store in a cool, dry place and keep all water out of the container. This scrub powder can keep up to 6 months.

MAKES 1 OUNCE SCRUB POWDER (ABOUT 20 APPLICATIONS)

1 tablespoon pure white tea leaves

6 tablespoons finely ground (colloidal) oatmeal

3 tablespoons rice flour

1 (1.5-ounce) airtight container

SPOTLESS GEL

Inspired by Origins' Super Spot Remover

MAKES 1 (0.5-OUNCE) SPOT TREATMENT (ABOUT 15–20 APPLICATIONS)

1 teaspoon grapeseed oil

2–6 drops tea tree essential oil

1 tablespoon aloe vera gel

1 (0.6-ounce) airtight container

Dreaming of a spotless face? The antibacterial tea tree oil in this homemade remedy is a natural alternative to the harsh ingredients sometimes found in acne treatments. The amount of tea tree oil you use in this recipe depends on your skin's sensitivity. If you have very sensitive skin, go for the smaller amount of oil.

Not a Fan of Tea Tree Oil?

If you've ever caught a whiff of tea tree oil, you know it comes with a distinct scent. I've gotten used to the smell, and it's still my favorite oil to fight acne. But if you really can't stand it, use lavender essential oil instead.

HOW TO MAKE:

1 Add grapeseed oil and essential oil to a small mixing bowl. Stir until the oils are evenly combined.

2 Add aloe vera gel and stir well until you get an even mixture.

3 Scoop the mixture into the container.

HOW TO USE:

Use this acne-fighting gel as part of your nighttime routine. Always use clean fingers or a clean cotton pad or swab when you dip into your container. After applying your face oil or moisturizer, dab a little bit of gel on top of any zits popping up. Avoid your eye area.

HOW TO STORE:

Store any leftover gel in the refrigerator and use within 3–5 days.

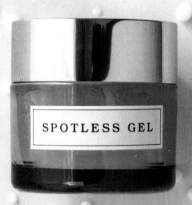

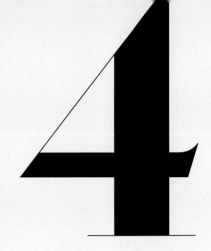

CHAPTER 4

MADE TO GLOW

Your warrior face. Your security blanket. Your bring-it-on look. A full face of makeup has many functions.

Now imagine that those products you love are actually hurting your skin. That became my reality. I developed eczema on my face, and no matter what beauty products I used to cover it up and treat it, nothing seemed to help. Then my dermatologist gave me some shocking information: the lip balms and lipsticks I was using to cover up my eczema breakouts were actually making it worse!

I had to rethink my entire makeup collection. Since I couldn't find any good hypoallergenic alternatives, I started making my own makeup products. The first item I ever made was a simple moisturizing lip balm. And I've never looked back since.

This chapter is dedicated to homemade makeup products like eye shadows and creams, lip balms and masks, and blushes and bronzers. With these handmade makeup items you can enhance your natural glow.

Essential Essential Oils

Of course essential oils smell amazing, but did you know that each essential oil has its own beauty benefits? Just a few drops can completely transform a recipe.

When you're new to essential oils, the choice might feel overwhelming. Here are my top picks for your starter kit; you'll see them a lot in the recipes of this book.

- **Geranium:** I love this essential oil for its sweet, floral scent. Use this oil in combination with other essential oils. This oil has a very noticeably stimulating scent, perfect if you want to combat negative thoughts or get rid of stress. It also has skin benefits. It's a good choice if you suffer from eczema or psoriasis, and this balancing oil works for acne-prone skin too.

- **Lavender:** Lavender essential oil is very versatile, making it a popular choice in many skincare recipes. This oil is said to have antibacterial and anti-inflammatory properties, making it ideal for both acne-prone and sensitive skin. But lavender essential oil is best known for its calming properties, helping you with anxiety and catching some beauty sleep.

- **Peppermint:** Peppermint is a very refreshing essential oil, as it can feel cooling on the skin. That makes it a perfect choice for a balm or lotion bar applied to aching, tired muscles. And I love it in a refreshing foot spray. Its stimulating scent can also help you wake up and focus. But use this powerful essential oil with caution on sensitive skin.

- **Tea tree:** Tea tree might not be the best-smelling essential oil and is often overlooked, but it has great skin benefits. This oil has been effectively used as an acne treatment, and it's praised for its antibacterial properties. I believe this oil is a must-have for people with acne-prone skin.

- **Ylang-ylang:** Made from the freshly picked flowers of the ylang-ylang tree, this essential oil has a floral, exotic scent. It is said to have a calming and relaxing effect, so it is a great choice for a body oil or a bath bomb. It can also be used for all skin types, as it's said to hydrate and soften the skin. Ylang-ylang oil has a very overpowering scent, so a little goes a long way. I love to combine this oil with lavender and geranium.

Always dilute an essential oil in a carrier oil before you apply it on your skin. Read more about the safe use of essential oils in Chapter 1.

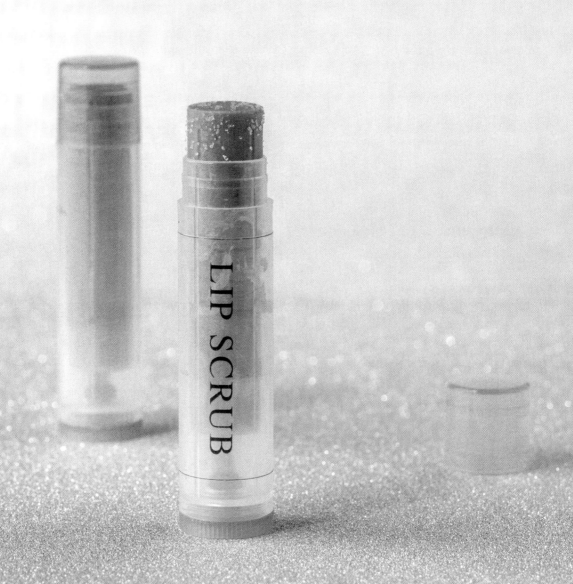

TWIST-UP LIP SCRUB

Inspired by Dior's Lip Sugar Scrub

A lip balm that doubles as a lip scrub?! This twist-up lip scrub will become your new go-to beauty essential on busy mornings.

HOW TO MAKE:

1 Slowly melt beeswax and shea butter in a double boiler over medium heat.

2 Add jojoba oil and stir until all the ingredients are combined.

3 Add cosmetic mica to the melted mixture. Stir to evenly distribute the color.

4 Add sugar and stir until it is evenly distributed throughout the mixture. Now you can take the double boiler off the heat.

5 Make sure the mechanism of each twist-up container is wound all the way down to the bottom. Carefully divide the mixture among the containers. Use a teaspoon to avoid spills. Leave to set 2–3 hours or until solid before use.

HOW TO USE:

To use, just pucker up and glide this dazzling duo over your lips. The sugar grains will scrub away any flakes, and the lip balm will leave your lips feeling moisturized. Gently buff away any leftover sugar grains with clean fingers. Now you're left with a beautiful, soft pink sheen.

HOW TO STORE:

Store in a cool, dry place up to 6 months.

MAKES 3 (0.15-OUNCE) LIP SCRUB BALMS

1 teaspoon white beeswax pellets

1 teaspoon shea butter

1 teaspoon jojoba oil

$\frac{1}{8}$ teaspoon pink cosmetic mica

$\frac{1}{2}$ teaspoon sugar

3 (0.15-ounce) twist-up containers

Stuck on Beeswax

Beeswax has a higher melting point than most butters and oils. That makes it harder to remove from utensils. Let your utensils soak in hot water first to melt the beeswax. Use this trick only for heatproof utensils, as you don't want your glass to burst or your plastic to melt!

ALL-IN-ONE STICK

Inspired by Nars' The Multiple

**MAKES 1 (0.6-OUNCE)
MOISTURIZING BALM**

½ tablespoon white beeswax pellets

1 tablespoon shea butter

½ tablespoon coconut oil

½ teaspoon cosmetic mica in color of your choice

1 (0.6-ounce) twist-up container

On your lips, your cheekbones, your collarbones, or all the way down your legs: use this all-natural solid lotion body balm to highlight your best features!

HOW TO MAKE:

1 Melt beeswax and shea butter in a double boiler over medium heat. Let them melt together until they're liquid.

2 Take the double boiler off the heat and add coconut oil. Stir the mixture until all ingredients are combined.

3 Add cosmetic mica and stir until the mixture is an even color.

4 Make sure the mechanism of the twist-up container is wound all the way down to the bottom. Carefully pour the mixture into the container. Use a small funnel to avoid spilling. Give this balm 2–3 hours to set before use.

HOW TO USE:

Apply an even layer of this multi-purpose balm on clean, dry skin.

HOW TO STORE:

Store in a cool, dry place up to 6 months.

BLUSH LIP GLOSS

Inspired by Tom Ford's Lip Lacquer

This long-lasting gloss leaves a pretty sheen while the oils moisturize your lips!

HOW TO MAKE:

1 Melt beeswax and coconut oil in a double boiler over medium heat. Stir occasionally until the mixture has melted together.

2 Take the double boiler off the heat and add castor oil. Stir well to combine.

3 Add cosmetic mica and stir until the color is evenly distributed.

4 Pour mixture into empty containers.

5 Wait 2–3 hours until it has set and is ready to use.

HOW TO USE:

1 Take a little bit of gloss out of the container using clean fingers or an applicator.

2 Apply an even layer on your lips. Repeat when the color and gloss start to fade.

HOW TO STORE:

Store in a cool, dry place out of direct sunlight up to 6 months.

MAKES 2 (0.3-OUNCE) LIP GLOSSES

$\frac{1}{2}$ **teaspoon beeswax pellets**

$\frac{1}{2}$ **tablespoon coconut oil**

1 tablespoon castor oil

$\frac{1}{4}$ **teaspoon cosmetic mica in color of your choice**

2 (0.3-ounce) containers or lip gloss applicators

BROWS GEL

Inspired by Anastasia Beverly Hills' Clear Brow Gel

MAKES 1 (0.6-OUNCE) BROW GEL

1 tablespoon aloe vera gel

1 teaspoon castor oil

1 (0.7-ounce) airtight container

Bushy brows, monobrow, or skinny brows: whichever style you're rocking, this all-natural gel will help keep your brows in shape. The castor oil will strengthen the hairs and add shine.

HOW TO MAKE:

1 Scoop aloe vera gel into a small mixing bowl. Add castor oil and stir until combined.

2 Scoop the gel into the airtight container.

HOW TO USE:

1 Dip a clean mascara wand in the container to get a little bit of gel on the brush.

2 Gently comb the hairs of your eyebrows. Give the gel a few seconds to air-dry.

HOW TO STORE:

Store this gel in the refrigerator up to 3–5 days.

COCOA BRONZER

Inspired by Too Faced's Chocolate Soleil Bronzer

This bronzer uses colors from Mother Nature. Achieve a natural, sun-kissed tint with deliciously smelling cinnamon and cocoa powder!

MAKES 1 (0.3-OUNCE) BRONZER

1 teaspoon arrowroot powder

2 teaspoons cocoa powder

1 teaspoon ground cinnamon

1/8 teaspoon gold cosmetic mica (optional)

1 (0.5-ounce) airtight container

High-proof (at least 70 percent) alcohol in a spray bottle (optional)

HOW TO MAKE:

1 Combine arrowroot powder, cocoa powder, ground cinnamon, and gold cosmetic mica, if using, in a small mixing bowl. Stir until the mixture has an even color. You can adjust the ratios until you get the color you like.

2 Scoop the loose powder into the container.

3 This step is optional but necessary if you want to turn the loose powder into a compact powder. Spray the top liberally with alcohol until it's soaked. Wait until the alcohol has evaporated completely before use. This might take 1 day.

HOW TO USE:

1 Dip a clean makeup brush into the container or swirl the brush over the compact powder. Tap any excess powder from the brush.

2 Apply a thin layer on parts of your face that can use a bit of bronzing.

HOW TO STORE:

Store in a cool, dry place up to 6 months.

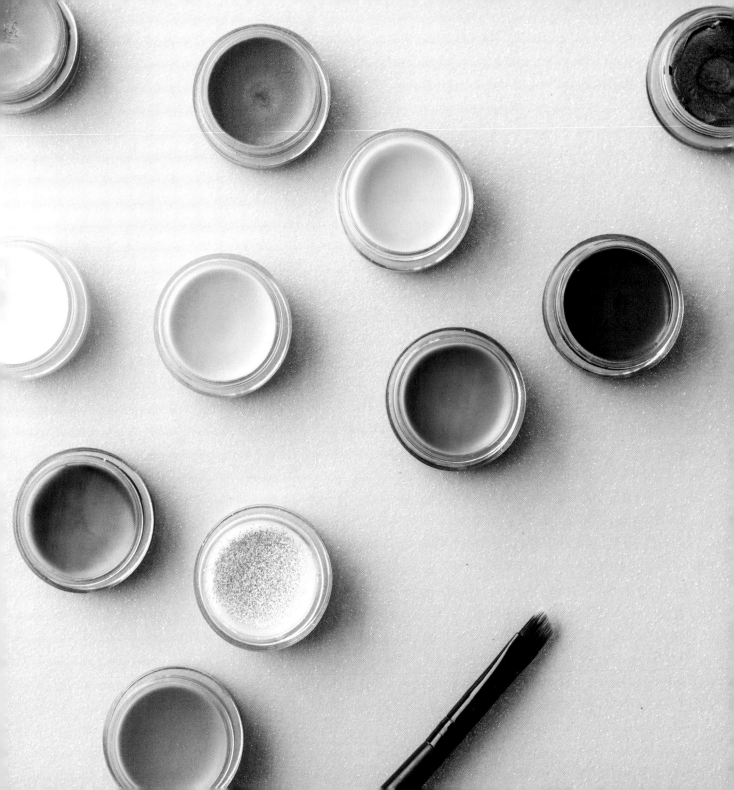

CREAMY EYE SHADOW

Inspired by Maybelline's Eyestudio ColorTattoo 24HR Cream Gel Eye Shadow

There are no limits to your imagination when you make your own eye shadows. You can add any color cosmetic mica you desire to this recipe so you can go for bold and make your eyes pop.

HOW TO MAKE:

1 Slowly melt beeswax in a double boiler over medium heat.

2 When beeswax starts to soften, add shea butter to the double boiler and let the ingredients melt together. Stir occasionally.

3 Add castor oil to the mixture once beeswax and shea butter turn to liquid.

4 Add cosmetic mica. Stir the mixture with a spoon to combine all the ingredients. Take the double boiler off the heat.

5 Divide the melted mixture evenly among the containers. Give your eye shadows 2–3 hours to set before use. Place covered in the refrigerator to quicken the cooling process.

HOW TO USE:

1 Dip a clean makeup brush into the container and swirl. Apply the eye shadow with even, gentle strokes on your eyelids.

2 This cream eye shadow works great on its own, or you can layer your favorite powder eye shadow on top for additional staying power.

MAKES 3 (0.25-OUNCE) EYE SHADOWS

1 teaspoon white beeswax pellets

2 teaspoons shea butter

2 teaspoons castor oil

2 teaspoons cosmetic mica in color of your choice

3 (0.3-ounce) containers

HOW TO STORE:

Store in a cool, dry place out of direct sunlight up to 6 months.

CLEAN MY BRUSHES KIT

Inspired by Sephora Collection's Purifying Brush Shampoo

MAKES 1 (1.7-OUNCE) BRUSH CLEANSER

1.2 ounces unscented liquid Castile soap

0.5 ounce olive oil

1 (2-ounce) airtight shampoo or pump bottle

3 drops tea tree essential oil

3 drops eucalyptus essential oil

A good makeup routine starts with the right tools. It's only natural that you should take just as much care of your makeup brushes as you do for the rest of your kit.

HOW TO MAKE:

1 Pour Castile soap and olive oil into the bottle. Use a small funnel to avoid spills.

2 Add essential oils.

3 Screw on the lid and shake to mix.

2 Pour or pump about 1 teaspoon of brush cleanser in a small dish or in the palm of your hand. Swirl the wet brush in the cleanser until it starts to foam.

3 Rinse the bristles thoroughly. Repeat if necessary.

HOW TO USE:

1 Hold your brush underneath a running tap until the bristles are soaked. Shake the bottle of brush cleaner vigorously before each use.

HOW TO STORE:

Store in a cool, dry place up to 6 months.

EYE COAT

Inspired by Laura Mercier's Eye Basics

The base of any good eye makeup is your primer. Coat your lids with this primer first to make your powder eyeshadow pop!

HOW TO MAKE:

1 Melt beeswax and mango butter in a double boiler over medium heat. Stir occasionally until the ingredients have melted. Add jojoba oil and stir to combine.

2 Stir in arrowroot powder. Keep stirring the mixture for a few minutes until the arrowroot powder has dissolved.

3 Add cosmetic mica and stir until the mixture is an even color. Take the double boiler off the heat.

4 Carefully divide the mixture between the containers. Use a small funnel to avoid spilling if you're using eye shadow applicators. Wait 5–8 hours for the mixture to set or until it's no longer runny. Place the containers covered in the refrigerator to quicken the cooling process.

HOW TO USE:

1 Use the applicator or a clean fingertip to pat a thin layer of eye primer onto your eyelid.

2 Give it a few seconds to dry. Use an eye shadow on top of the eye primer for long-lasting color.

MAKES 2 (0.25-OUNCE) EYE PRIMERS

1 teaspoon beeswax pellets

1 teaspoon mango butter

2 teaspoons jojoba oil

1 teaspoon arrowroot powder

1/4 teaspoon cosmetic mica in color of your choice (optional)

2 (0.3-ounce) airtight containers or cream eye shadow applicators

HOW TO STORE:

Store in a cool, dry place out of direct sunlight up to 6 months. Don't use this eye primer if the balm has become runny due to warm temperatures.

INSTANT LIP SCRUB

Inspired by Burt's Bees' Conditioning Lip Scrub

MAKES 1 INSTANT LIP SCRUB

1 teaspoon sugar

1 teaspoon honey

Looking for an instant lip treatment? Head over to the kitchen. You need only two simple ingredients to instantly soften your flaky lips.

HOW TO MAKE:

1 Scoop sugar into a small mixing bowl.

2 Add honey and stir, stir, stir!

HOW TO USE:

1 Apply a thick layer of this homemade lip scrub all over your lips. Resist the urge to lick it off. Make small circular motions with your fingers to massage your lips.

2 Once your lips feel soft, rinse off the lip scrub with lukewarm water.

HOW TO STORE:

This lip scrub is meant for a single, immediate use.

FAIRY DIRT POWDER

Inspired by Active Wow's Activated Coconut Charcoal Powder Natural Teeth Whitening

Can't survive without that morning cup of coffee? Sippin' tea like you're the queen? This powder will make your teeth sparkling white again!

MAKES 0.6 OUNCE POWDER (ABOUT 9 APPLICATIONS)

3 tablespoons activated charcoal

1 tablespoon coconut oil

1 (0.7-ounce) airtight container

HOW TO MAKE:

1 Scoop activated charcoal into a small mixing bowl.

2 Melt coconut oil using a double boiler over medium heat. Or heat coconut oil in a heatproof bowl in the microwave on a low setting (650 watts or lower) for 1 minute.

3 Drizzle melted coconut oil over charcoal. Stir vigorously to make sure charcoal is evenly combined with the oil. Place mixture into the container.

HOW TO USE:

1 Scoop 1/3 teaspoon powder out of the container with a spoon.

2 Dip a clean toothbrush in the powder, then wet the toothbrush. Softly brush your teeth with the mixture.

3 Rinse your mouth until most of the black is removed from your teeth. Now brush your teeth as you normally would.

4 If you worry about the powder being too abrasive for your teeth, you can also swish it. Dilute 1/4 teaspoon powder in 1 tablespoon water and swirl the mixture around your mouth. I don't recommend using this teeth powder daily. Save it for special occasions.

HOW TO STORE:

Store in a cool, dry place and keep all water out of the container. This powder can keep up to 6 months.

CLEANSING BALM

Inspired by Goop by Juice Beauty's Luminous Melting Cleanser

MAKES 1 (2.5-OUNCE) BALM

0.2 ounce beeswax pellets

1.5 ounces shea butter

0.4 ounce coconut oil

0.4 ounce olive oil

1 (3-ounce) airtight container

I love to use a cleansing balm when I want to remove a full face of makeup. This balm is the perfect choice for dry skin types. Use it to remove stubborn waterproof makeup or just to cleanse your pretty face.

HOW TO MAKE:

1 Melt beeswax, shea butter, and coconut oil in a double boiler over medium heat. Stir occasionally until the ingredients have melted.

2 Take the double boiler off the heat and stir in olive oil.

3 Pour the melted mixture into the airtight container. Let the balm set 2–3 hours before use. Place covered in the refrigerator to quicken the cooling process.

HOW TO USE:

1 Dampen your face with warm water. Take a chickpea-sized amount of balm out of the container using a spoon, a spatula, or clean, dry fingers.

2 Apply the balm to your face and gently massage your face with your fingertips.

3 You can use this balm to carefully remove eye makeup too. Just make sure you don't get any balm in your eyes.

4 Use a warm, damp washcloth to wipe away the balm and makeup gunk. Follow with a mild toner or flower water to remove all traces of the cleansing balm.

HOW TO STORE:

Store in a cool, dry place and keep all water out of the container. This balm can keep up to 6 months.

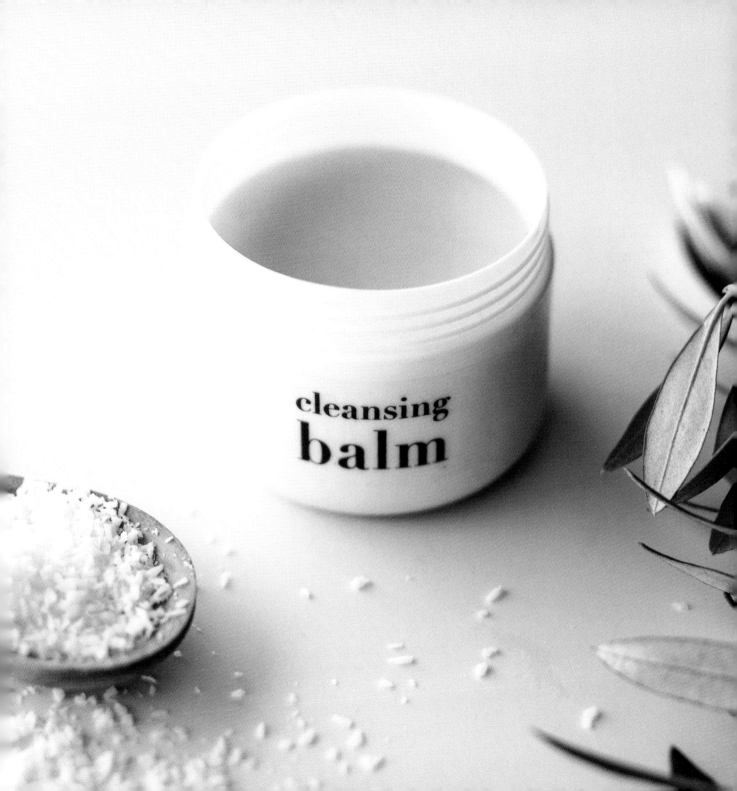

JIGGLY HIGHLIGHTER

Inspired by Farsáli's Jelly Beam Illuminator/Highlighter

MAKES 1 (1-OUNCE) HIGHLIGHTER

¼ teaspoon beeswax pellets

3 tablespoons jojoba oil

1½ tablespoons arrowroot powder

1 teaspoon gold or pearl cosmetic mica

1 (1.5-ounce) airtight container

This gooey, gel-like highlighter turns to powder on your skin!

HOW TO MAKE:

1 Slowly melt beeswax in a double boiler over medium heat.

2 Add jojoba oil and stir until beeswax has dissolved into jojoba oil.

3 Add arrowroot powder and stir until the powder has dissolved completely.

4 Add cosmetic mica and stir until the mica has colored the mixture evenly. You can add gold or pearl mica, or mix both to create your own custom color.

5 Take the double boiler off the heat and pour the mixture into the airtight container. Let it set 2–3 hours before use. Place covered in the refrigerator to quicken the cooling process.

HOW TO USE:

1 Dip a clean, dry makeup brush in the container to coat the bristles with the highlighter.

2 Apply a thin layer where the light naturally hits your face, like your cheekbones. Blend with the brush or use clean fingers.

HOW TO STORE:

Store in a cool, dry place out of direct sunlight up to 6 months.

LASH BOOSTER

Inspired by Shiseido's Full Lash Serum

You take care of your skin, your lips, and your brows. But what about your lashes? This glossy oil will coat your lashes, making them look thick and healthy. This oil can be used on your eyebrows too!

MAKES 1 APPLICATION

1 drop castor oil

1 cotton pad

HOW TO MAKE:

Place drop of castor oil onto the cotton pad. Carefully fold the pad so castor oil spreads evenly.

HOW TO STORE:

This lash booster is meant for a single, immediate use. Use a new cotton pad for each application.

HOW TO USE:

1 Close your eyes and carefully pat the castor oil onto your lashes. Make sure you don't get any oil in your eye.

2 Wipe away any excess oil on your eyelids and underneath your eyes with micellar water, a mild toner, or a flower water.

LIP BALM IN A TIN

Inspired by Burt's Bees' Beeswax Lip Balm

MAKES 2 (0.4-OUNCE) LIP BALMS

0.2 ounce white beeswax pellets

0.4 ounce shea butter

0.2 ounce coconut oil

1 drop peppermint essential oil

2 (0.4-ounce) aluminum tin lip balm containers

Mind Your Mint

Peppermint, although wildly cooling and refreshing, is a very overpowering essential oil. So please use it with care on sensitive skin.

Who knew such a small tin could pack such a refreshing punch? One drop of peppermint essential oil is all it takes to get that minty fresh, tingling feeling on your lips!

HOW TO MAKE:

1 Slowly melt beeswax, shea butter, and coconut oil in a double boiler over medium heat.

2 Take the double boiler off the heat and let the mixture cool down a bit. Add peppermint essential oil to the melted ingredients. Stir to combine.

3 Divide the mixture between the lip balm tins. Give the lip balms 2–3 hours to set before use. Place covered in the refrigerator to quicken the cooling process.

HOW TO USE:

When your lips are in need of some serious refreshment, just twist your tin open, swirl a clean finger or lip brush over the lip balm, pout your lips, and apply a thin layer all over.

HOW TO STORE:

Throw a tin in your bag and you'll never find yourself in a lip care emergency. Keep in mind, though, that the balms might melt at high temperatures. These minty lip balms can keep up to 6 months.

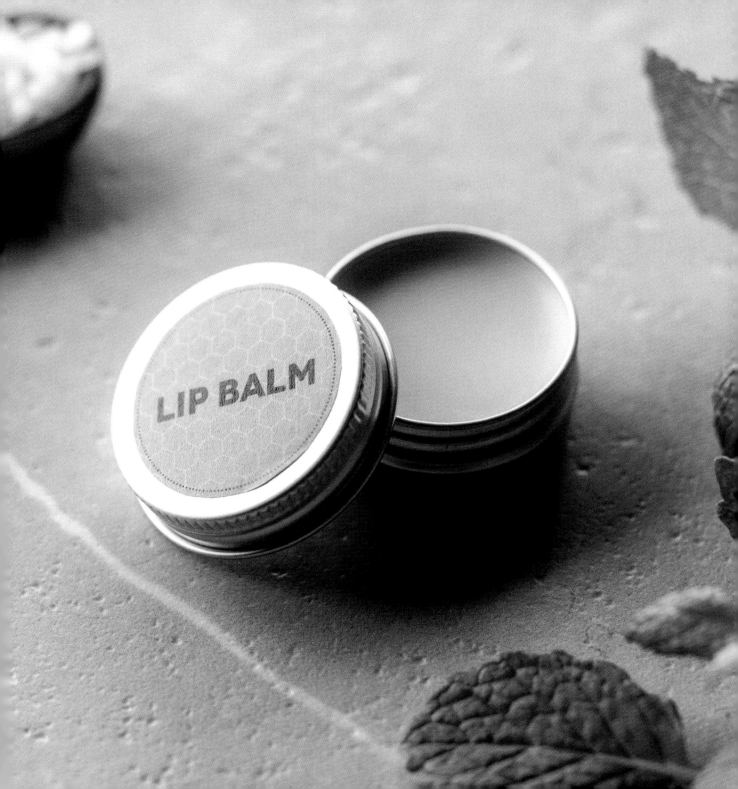

LIP BASE

Inspired by MAC's Prep + Prime Lip

MAKES 3 (0.15-OUNCE) LIP BALMS

1 tablespoon white beeswax pellets

1 tablespoon sweet almond oil

3 (0.15-ounce) twist-up containers

To make sure your lipstick won't bleed or fade, you need a solid base. This waxy lip base will make sure your lip shade stays put.

HOW TO MAKE:

1 Melt beeswax in a double boiler over medium heat.

2 Once beeswax starts to melt, add sweet almond oil to the double boiler and stir to combine.

3 Divide the melted mixture among the containers. Let set 2–3 hours or until solid before use.

HOW TO USE:

1 For perfect, long-lasting color, start with scrubbed, dry lips.

2 Apply a thin layer of lip base. Make sure to coat along the edges of your lips as well.

3 Apply a layer of your favorite lip shade on top. Add more layers of lipstick until you reach the desired color and consistency.

HOW TO STORE:

Store in a cool, dry place up to 6 months.

SET MY MAKEUP POWDER

Inspired by Laura Mercier's Translucent Loose Setting Powder

A makeup powder stops your forehead from turning into a disco ball midway through your day. This simple DIY recipe makes an oil-absorbing face powder in an instant.

MAKES 0.3 OUNCE FACE POWDER

3 tablespoons arrowroot powder

1 teaspoon bentonite clay

1 (1-ounce) airtight container

HOW TO MAKE:

Scoop arrowroot powder and bentonite clay into the airtight container. Put on the lid and shake to combine the ingredients. Wait until the powder has settled to the bottom before opening the container again.

HOW TO USE:

1 Dip a clean makeup brush in your container. Tap off any excess. A little goes a very long way with this powder!

2 Sweep the brush across your face using circular motions, leaving a thin layer on your skin.

HOW TO STORE:

Store in a cool, dry place up to 3 months.

Spice It Up

Customize the color of your face powder by adding a dash of hibiscus, beetroot, ground cinnamon, or cocoa powder. Combine different colors until you have your own custom blend!

MAKEUP OIL CLEANSER

Inspired by MAC's Cleanse Off Oil

**MAKES 1 (2.1-OUNCE)
MAKEUP CLEANSER**

1 (2.5-ounce) pump or flip-cap bottle

1.2 ounces olive oil

0.6 ounce jojoba oil

0.3 ounce evening primrose oil

10 drops vitamin E oil

Simple olive oil and jojoba oil work together to remove even the most stubborn waterproof makeup. The evening primrose oil gives this cleanser an extra anti-inflammatory kick, perfect if you're suffering from eczema or acne. You might be surprised that this cleanser is loved by almost all skin types. Yes, oily skin too!

HOW TO MAKE:

1 Unscrew the lid from your pump or flip-cap bottle. Insert a small funnel into the opening of the bottle to avoid spilling.

2 Pour olive oil, jojoba oil, and evening primrose oil through the funnel.

3 Remove the funnel and add vitamin E oil.

4 Screw the top back on and shake the bottle vigorously to mix all the ingredients.

HOW TO USE:

1 You may have heard of the oil cleansing method before. The cleansing oils dissolve the oils present in your makeup and make the gunk slide right off your face.

2 Pour about ½ tablespoon Makeup Oil Cleanser into the palm of your hand.

3 With clean fingers apply the cleanser on your dry face. Move it around with your fingertips to help remove your makeup. You can use this for eye makeup, too, but be very careful not to get the cleanser in your eyes.

4 Remove the cleanser and makeup gunk with a damp wash cloth or cotton wool pad.

5 Follow with a mild toner or flower water to remove any remaining traces of cleanser.

HOW TO STORE:

Evening primrose oil has a short shelf life. That's why we're adding vitamin E oil. Store this cleanser in a cool, dry place out of direct sunlight and use within 3 months.

MANGO LIP MASK

Inspired by Kiehl's Buttermask for Lips

**MAKES 1 (0.3-OUNCE)
LIP MASK BALM**

1 teaspoon mango butter

1 teaspoon coconut oil

1 (0.4-ounce) airtight container

Just when you think you've seen it all, here's a mask for smooth, touchable lips. You might see a slight color difference between your DIY version and the product that inspired it because this recipe uses only two simple, natural ingredients.

HOW TO MAKE:

1 Melt mango butter and coconut oil in a double boiler over medium heat.

2 Stir occasionally until the ingredients have melted and combined. Take the double boiler off the heat and pour the melted mixture into the container. Wait 2–3 hours or until it's solid before use.

HOW TO USE:

1 Use clean, dry fingers or a lip brush to apply a thin layer all over your lips before you go to bed, and you'll wake up the next morning with silky, soft lips.

2 You can also use this as an instant treatment. Apply a thick layer on your lips and let sit about 10 minutes. Wipe away the excess.

HOW TO STORE:

Store in a cool, dry place out of direct sunlight up to 6 months.

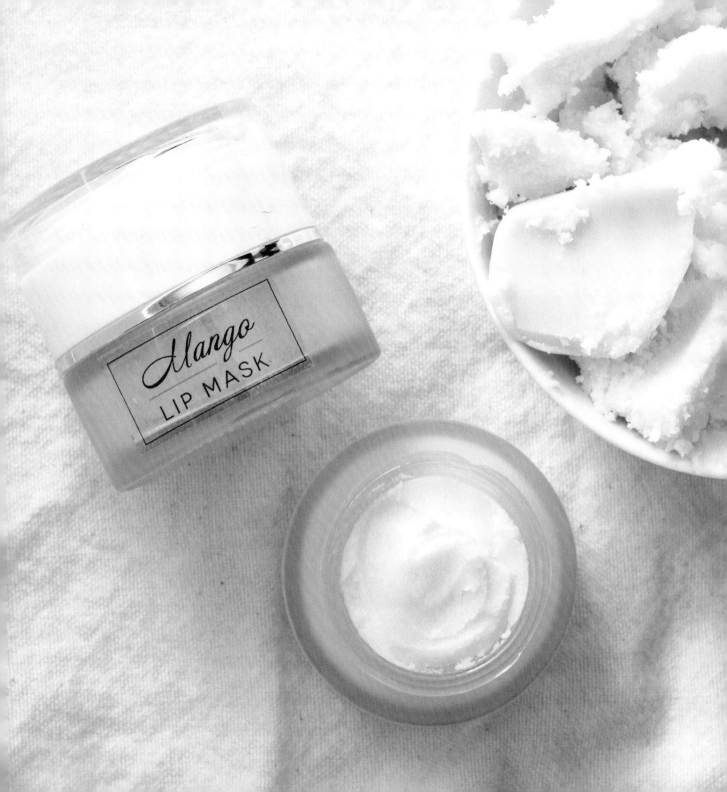

TINTED LIP BUTTER

Inspired by Maybelline's Baby Lips Moisturizing Lip Balm

MAKES 3 (0.15-OUNCE) LIP BALMS

1 teaspoon white beeswax pellets

1 teaspoon shea butter

1 teaspoon mango butter

1 teaspoon coconut oil

$\frac{1}{8}$ teaspoon cosmetic mica in color of your choice

3 (0.15-ounce) twist-up lip balm containers

This homemade lip treat is just as moisturizing, softening, and shimmery as many store-bought balms!

HOW TO MAKE:

1 Combine beeswax, shea butter, mango butter, and coconut oil in a double boiler over medium heat. Let them slowly melt together.

2 Add cosmetic mica to the melted mixture. Stir to mix the melted ingredients and to evenly distribute the color.

3 Make sure the twist-up mechanism of each container is wound all the way down to the bottom. Take the double boiler off the heat and carefully divide the melted mixture between the containers using a teaspoon. A small funnel can help avoid spilling.

4 Let the lip balms set 2–3 hours. Put them covered in the refrigerator if you want to quicken the cooling process.

HOW TO USE:

When your lips can use a pick-me-up, glide this lip balm over your lips. The all-natural ingredients will soothe and moisturize your skin. And the mica will leave a subtle sheen!

HOW TO STORE:

Store in a cool, dry place up to 6 months. These are perfect to keep in your emergency makeup kit or your handbag. Just be careful with hot temperatures, as the natural butters and oil might melt slightly.

VEGANILLA LIP BALM

Inspired by Hurraw!'s Vanilla Bean Lip Balm

This vegan lip balm is infused with vanilla to make your lips smell and feel amazing!

HOW TO MAKE:

1 Melt cocoa butter using a double boiler over medium heat. Or melt cocoa butter in a heatproof container in the microwave on a low setting (650 watts or lower) using 1-minute intervals until cocoa butter has melted.

2 Once cocoa butter has melted, take the double boiler off the heat or take the container out of the microwave.

3 Add vanilla-infused coconut oil and stir until coconut oil has dissolved.

4 Make sure the twist-up mechanism of each lip balm container is wound all the way down to the bottom. Carefully divide the mixture among the containers. Use a small funnel to avoid spilling.

5 Leave the balms to set 2–3 hours or until hard. Place them covered in the refrigerator to quicken the cooling process.

HOW TO USE:

Glide this balm over your lips and enjoy the sweet, chocolatey scent of cocoa butter and vanilla!

HOW TO STORE:

Store the balms in a cool, dry place up to 6 months. Keep in mind that the balms might melt slightly at high temperatures.

MAKES 3 (0.2-OUNCE) LIP BALMS

2 tablespoons cocoa butter

1 teaspoon vanilla-infused coconut oil (see Shiny Body Oil recipe in Chapter 5)

3 (0.2-ounce) lip balm containers

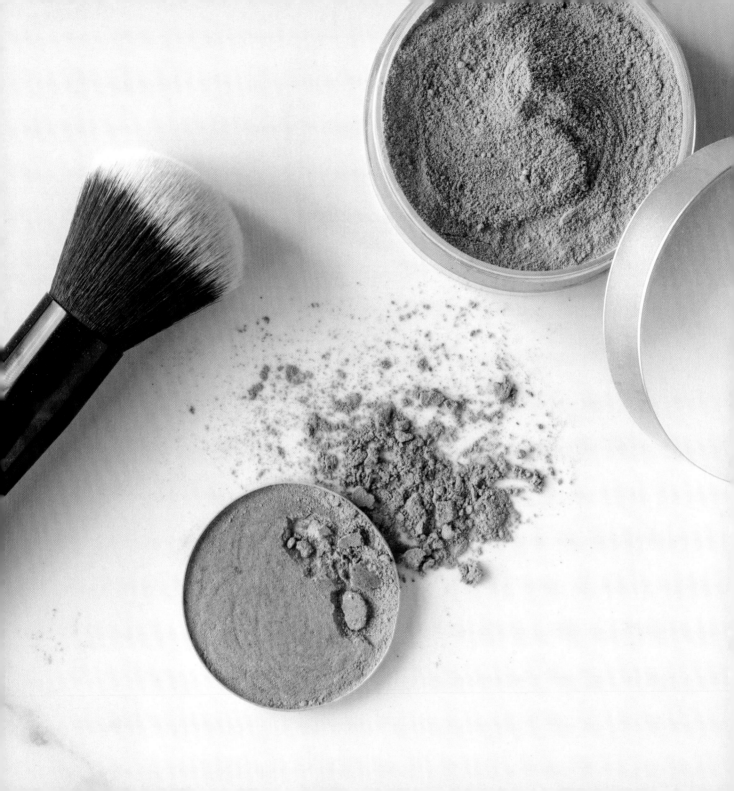

SUPERWOMAN BLUSH

Inspired by Tarte's Amazonian Clay 12-Hour Blush

This all-natural recipe makes a gorgeous coral blush that's a perfect match for my complexion. Add more arrowroot powder for a lighter color, or more beetroot or hibiscus powder for a deeper pink color. You can have your own custom shade in no time!

MAKES 1 (0.4-OUNCE) BLUSH POWDER

1 tablespoon arrowroot powder

½ teaspoon pink clay

½ teaspoon beetroot or hibiscus powder

1 (0.5-ounce) airtight container

High-proof (at least 70 percent) alcohol in a spray bottle

HOW TO MAKE:

1 Scoop arrowroot powder, pink clay, and beetroot or hibiscus powder into a small mixing bowl. Stir until the powder has an even color.

2 Scoop loose powder into the container, pressing and packing it down as you go.

3 This step will turn this blush powder into a compact powder: Spray the mixture liberally with alcohol until it's soaked. Wait until alcohol has evaporated before use. This might take 1 day.

HOW TO USE:

Swirl a clean makeup brush over the compact powder. Swipe the brush across the apples of your cheeks.

HOW TO STORE:

Store in a cool, dry place up to 6 months.

Keep It Loose

You also have the option of leaving this blush as a loose powder and not pressing it into a compact powder. To leave the blush loose, simply place the powder in your storage container without packing it down and don't spray the mixture with the alcohol. Then when you are ready to use simply dip your makeup brush in the loose powder, tap off any excess, and sweep it onto the apples of your cheeks.

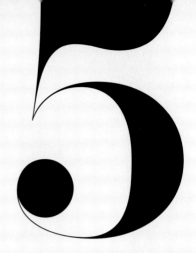

CHAPTER 5
BODY LOVE

Just like the skin on your face can act out, so can the skin on other parts of your body. Dry patches, those bumps on the backs of your arms, dimples on your thighs...you name it. Although we should worry less about appearances and embrace what Mother Nature gave us, it helps to know there are natural remedies that can help with those problems.

In this chapter you'll find beauty recipes for everything from your shoulders all the way down to the tips of your toes. Your skin is the largest organ of your body, so you'd better treat it in the best way you can! A luxurious body scrub or a nice body cream can do wonders for your body and mind. And how about those hands and feet that do so much work for you? It's about time you give your body some love!

LET'S BREW AN OIL

We've already discussed the great benefits of plant-based oils, but what if you could make them even better? When you infuse an oil with dried herbs or flowers, you basically get a super oil. When you make an infused oil, you extract some of the powerful properties of the herbs and flowers so they can be used in your homemade skincare products. Make sure you use dried ingredients, as we don't want to introduce water to the oil! Popular flowers to infuse oils with are dried chamomile, calendula, and lavender flowers. We'll also be using vanilla- and coffee-infused oils for some of the recipes in this book.

There are two ways to infuse oils: the "cold" method and the "hot" method.

Cold Infusion

1 To begin we'll need a perfectly clean and dry airtight container.

2 Add the dry ingredients (dried flowers, for example) to the container. Top with a carrier oil.

3 Close the container and make sure no water, air, or other contaminants can get to the oil. Store the container in a dark place at room temperature. Let the oil infuse about 6–8 weeks.

4 Strain the oil through a cheesecloth, a coffee filter, or a very fine-mesh sieve. Strain again if necessary until there's only oil left.

Can't wait 6 weeks? Here's a method that takes only a few hours. For this you'll need your double boiler.

Hot Infusion

1 Fill your double boiler with your dry ingredient(s) (aka what you'll be infusing your oil with). Bring the water underneath to a simmer.

2 Top the dry ingredient(s) with the carrier oil of your choice until it's completely covered.

3 Allow the mixture to infuse 2–6 hours while the water is kept to a simmer. Stir approximately every 20 minutes. Some of the water might evaporate. Pour extra water into the bottom saucepan to make sure the oil stays heated.

4 Strain the oil through a cheesecloth, a coffee filter, or a very fine-mesh sieve. Strain again if necessary until there's only oil left.

5 Repeat the whole process with the same oil and fresh dry ingredients if you want a more concentrated, double-infused oil.

There are several recipes in this book that use infused oils, so look back to these pages when you need the techniques to make them.

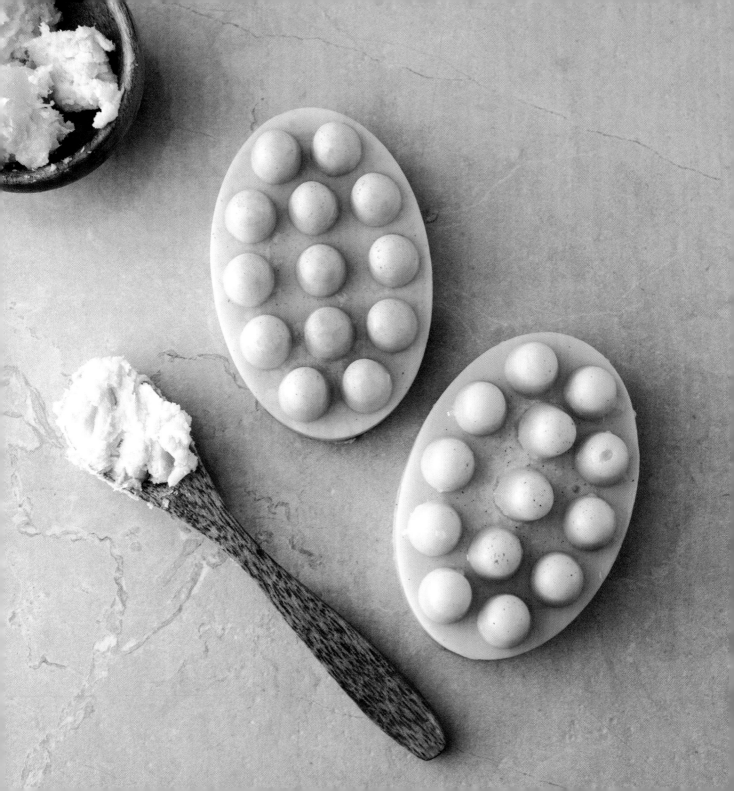

RUB BAR

Inspired by Lush's Therapy Massage Bar: Organic Neroli and Lavender Bar

This easy-to-make lotion bar doubles as a massage bar. Adjust the amount of essential oil you use based on your skin sensitivity and how subtle you want the scent.

MAKES 2 (1.75-OUNCE) LOTION BARS

2.7 ounces cocoa butter

0.8 ounce shea butter

10–15 drops essential oil of your choice

2 (1.75-ounce) oval-shaped silicone molds

HOW TO MAKE:

1 Slowly melt cocoa butter and shea butter in a double boiler over medium heat. Stir occasionally until butters are combined.

2 Take the double boiler off the heat and let the mixture sit a few minutes to cool. Add essential oil. Stir all the ingredients together until the oil is evenly distributed in the mixture.

3 Divide the mixture evenly between the molds. Give the bars 5–8 hours to set. Place the molds covered in the refrigerator to quicken the cooling process.

4 Pop the bars out of the molds once they're done and store them in an airtight container until you're ready to use them.

HOW TO USE:

After a nice shower or a long bath, run this Rub Bar over your dry skin. Use your hands to massage the butters into your skin.

HOW TO STORE:

Store your lotion bars in an airtight container in a cool, dry place up to 6 months.

Double the Rub

You could also add some coffee beans, adzuki beans, or jojoba beads to your lotion bar for an extra massage. Before you pour the mixture into the molds, put a few dry beans or beads at the bottom of the molds. Pour the mixture on top and let the bars cool as instructed.

BUTTER ME UP SCRUB

Inspired by L'Occitane's Shea Butter One-Minute Hand Scrub

MAKES 1 (6.8-OUNCE) HAND SCRUB

0.6 ounce shea butter

0.8 ounce coconut oil

1.4 ounces sweet almond oil

4 ounces sugar

1 (7-ounce) airtight container

This rich and creamy scrub moisturizes while it scrubs away flaky skin. The result: velvety soft, touchable hands!

HOW TO MAKE:

1 Melt shea butter in a double boiler over medium heat. Or melt shea butter in a heatproof container in the microwave on a low setting (650 watts or lower) using 1-minute intervals. Stir in between until the shea butter has melted.

2 Take the double boiler off the heat or take the container out of the microwave. Add coconut oil and stir to combine the ingredients.

3 Add almond oil and stir everything together.

4 Add sugar to a large mixing bowl. Carefully add the melted mixture to the sugar. Stir to mix the ingredients.

5 Scoop the mixture into the airtight container.

HOW TO USE:

1 Use a clean spoon or clean, dry hands to scoop about 1 teaspoon out of the container.

2 Gently rub the mixture between your hands, scrubbing your palms, fingers, and the backs of your hands.

3 Rinse off with plenty of water.

HOW TO STORE:

Store in a cool, dry place and keep all water out of the container. This hand scrub can keep up to 3 months.

COCOA SPREAD

Inspired by The Body Shop's Cocoa Body Butter

Cocoa butter leaves a protective layer on your skin, making this the perfect indulgent body balm!

MAKES 1 (3.5-OUNCE) BODY BALM

1.5 ounces cocoa butter

1 ounce jojoba oil

1 ounce sweet almond oil

1 (4-ounce) airtight container

HOW TO MAKE:

1 Melt cocoa butter in a double boiler over medium heat.

2 Once cocoa butter has melted, take the double boiler off the heat. Pour melted cocoa butter into a large mixing bowl and add jojoba oil and sweet almond oil. Stir the ingredients together until the oils are incorporated.

3 Set aside the mixture to thicken. Place it covered in the refrigerator for about 50 minutes to quicken the cooling process. Take the mixing bowl out before the mixture starts to become firm.

4 Whip the mixture with an electric whisk or mixer starting at a low setting. Keep whipping until the balm has a fluffy consistency.

5 Scoop the whipped body balm into the airtight container.

HOW TO USE:

1 Take a tiny amount out of the container. A little goes a very long way with this balm!

2 Spread it out evenly over your body. Massage it into the skin with your hands. Wait a few minutes for the balm to sink into your skin.

HOW TO STORE:

Store in a cool, dry place out of direct sunlight up to 6 months.

CREAM CORPORELLE

Inspired by La Mer's The Body Crème

MAKES 1 (4.8-OUNCE) BODY BUTTER

1.6 ounces avocado butter

1.8 ounces coconut oil

1.4 ounces grapeseed oil

25 drops vitamin E oil

1 (5-ounce) airtight container or pump bottle

It's fluffy, it's creamy, and it moisturizes your skin like crazy. It's whipped body butter!

HOW TO MAKE:

1 Melt avocado butter in a double boiler over medium heat. Or melt avocado butter in a heatproof container in the microwave on a low setting (650 watts or lower) using 1-minute intervals. Stir in between until butter has melted.

2 Take the double boiler off the heat or take the container out of the microwave. Stir in coconut oil and grapeseed oil until dissolved.

3 Pour the mixture into a large mixing bowl and wait until the ingredients start to thicken. Place the mixing bowl covered in the refrigerator for about 50 minutes to quicken the cooling process.

4 When the mixture has thickened to a pudding-like consistency, add vitamin E oil.

5 Carefully whip the mixture using an electric whisk or mixer at a low setting. Keep whipping until the mixture has a fluffy consistency.

6 Transfer whipped body butter to the airtight container or pump bottle.

HOW TO USE:

1 Use this whipped butter on (very) dry skin. Use a spoon, a spatula, or clean, dry hands to scoop a pea-sized amount out of the container at a time. A little goes a long way with this body butter!

2 Spread the butter over your body and massage it in with your hands. Give your skin a few minutes to absorb the butter.

HOW TO STORE:

Store in a cool, dry place out of direct sunlight and keep all water out of the container. This body butter can keep up to 3 months.

HEAL BALM

Inspired by Earth Therapeutics' Cracked Heel Repair

MAKES 1 (3.5-OUNCE) BALM

1.7 ounces cocoa butter

0.5 ounce beeswax

0.8 ounce avocado butter

0.5 ounce avocado oil

15 drops tea tree essential oil

1 (3.5-ounce) stick container

This balm does more than heal cracked feet. Rub it on your elbows, knees, or any part of your body that suffers from rough patches of skin.

HOW TO MAKE:

1 Combine cocoa butter, beeswax, and avocado butter in a double boiler over medium heat. Stir occasionally until all the ingredients are melted.

2 Take the double boiler off the heat and stir in avocado oil.

3 Add tea tree essential oil. Stir well to combine all the ingredients.

4 Make sure the twist-up mechanism of your stick container is wound all the way down to the bottom. Pour the mixture into the container. Give the balm 5–8 hours to set before putting the cap on. Place the container covered in the refrigerator to quicken the cooling process.

HOW TO USE:

Take the cap off the container and glide the balm over any rough patches of skin. Use clean fingers to massage the balm into the skin. Always make sure to put the lid back on.

HOW TO STORE:

Store in a cool, dry place out of direct sunlight up to 6 months.

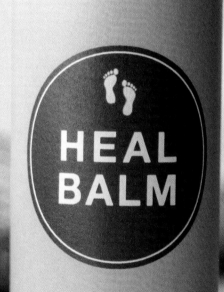

CUTICLE CUDDLE CREAM

Inspired by Burt's Bees' Lemon Butter Cuticle Cream

MAKES 2 (0.75-OUNCE) CUTICLE CREAMS

0.1 ounce beeswax pellets

0.6 ounce cocoa butter

0.8 ounce sweet almond oil

4 drops lemon essential oil

2 (1-ounce) containers

Lemon Sensitivity

Citrus essential oils like lemon and lime are considered phototoxic oils. This means they can cause sensitivity to the sun on the areas where you apply them. Avoid direct sunlight up to 12 hours after application. You could also swap the lemon for lemongrass essential oil instead.

Although often overlooked, your cuticles are an important part of your nails. So don't forget to give those cuticles some love!

HOW TO MAKE:

1 Melt beeswax and cocoa butter in a double boiler over medium heat.

2 Take the double boiler off the heat once wax and butter are melted. Add sweet almond oil and stir until all ingredients are well combined.

3 Add lemon essential oil and stir until the drops are spread evenly throughout the mixture.

4 Divide the mixture between the containers. Let set 2–3 hours before putting on the lids.

HOW TO USE:

1 When your cuticles are in need of a cuddle, it's time to bring out the cream. Rub a clean, dry finger over the cream to melt some of it.

2 Use your finger to apply a thin layer all around your nails. Massage it in for a real spa feeling.

HOW TO STORE:

Store in a cool, dry place out of direct sunlight up to 6 months.

ECZEMA ERASER BALM

Inspired by Aveeno's Eczema Therapy Itch Relief Balm

This luxurious balm is a treat for your skin! Use it for dry, itchy patches—for example, if you're suffering from eczema or psoriasis.

MAKES 1 (3.5-OUNCE) LOTION BALM

2.5 ounces shea butter

0.5 ounce chamomile- or calendula-infused sweet almond oil

0.5 ounce oat oil

1 (4-ounce) airtight container

HOW TO MAKE:

1 Melt shea butter in a double boiler over medium heat. Or melt shea butter in a heatproof container in the microwave on a low setting (650 watts or lower) using 1-minute intervals. Stir shea butter between intervals until it has completely melted.

2 Pour melted shea butter into a large mixing bowl. Add infused sweet almond oil and oat oil. Stir the ingredients together until combined.

3 Set aside the mixing bowl or place it covered in the refrigerator for about 50 minutes until the mixture starts to thicken.

4 Carefully whip the mixture with an electric whisk using the lowest setting. Keep whipping until the mixture develops a creamy "frosting" consistency.

5 Scoop the mixture into the airtight container.

HOW TO USE:

Apply a tiny amount of balm on any dry patches of skin and gently massage it in with your fingertips. Repeat as often as necessary.

HOW TO STORE:

Store in a cool, dry place up to 6 months.

How to Make Chamomile- or Calendula-Infused Sweet Almond Oil

To infuse sweet almond oil with dried chamomile or calendula flowers, follow the instructions at the beginning of this chapter. Infuse ½ cup sweet almond oil with about ¼ cup dried chamomile or calendula flowers. After measuring for your recipe, keep the leftover oil in an airtight container for up 6 months. With this infused oil you can also make the Salad Face Mask in Chapter 2 and the Floral Soap in Chapter 3.

FRAPPUCCINO BODY SCRUB

Inspired by Frank Body's Express-O Scrub

MAKES 1 (9.5-OUNCE) WHIPPED BODY SCRUB

1 ounce shea butter

2 ounces coconut oil

2 ounces cane sugar

2.5 ounces fine sea salt

2 ounces ground coffee beans

1 teaspoon (0.1 ounce) ground cinnamon

1 (10-ounce) airtight container

This rich body scrub exfoliates and moisturizes your skin at the same time!

HOW TO MAKE:

1 Melt shea butter in a double boiler over medium heat. Or melt shea butter in a heatproof container in the microwave on a low setting (650 watts or lower) using 1-minute intervals. Stir between intervals until shea butter has melted.

2 Take the double boiler off the heat or take the container out of the microwave. Add coconut oil and stir until oil has dissolved.

3 Pour the mixture into a large mixing bowl. Place the bowl covered in the refrigerator for 50 minutes to let it thicken. Take it out before it has set.

4 Carefully whip the thickened mixture with an electric whisk or mixer on a low setting until it starts to look like creamy frosting.

5 Add sugar, salt, ground coffee beans, and ground cinnamon to the mixing bowl. Carefully mix the ingredients together with a spoon until combined.

6 Scoop the body scrub into the airtight container.

HOW TO USE:

1 Scoop about 1–2 tablespoons whipped body scrub out of the container using a spoon or clean, dry fingers. Take this with you to the shower.

2 Gently massage the whipped scrub onto your wet skin. Rinse it off. Follow with soap to rinse off every last bit of scrub.

3 Use this body scrub once or twice a week. Oils can make your bathtub or shower floor slippery, so don't forget to clean up after you are done!

HOW TO STORE:

Store in a cool, dry place and keep all water out of the container. This body scrub can keep up to 3 months.

What about Used Coffee Grounds?

Used coffee grounds contain water, so never use them in your premade scrubs. But they do make the best frugal instant face and body scrub! Mix equal parts used coffee grounds and olive oil right before you plan to use it. Take the mixture with you in the shower and use it to gently scrub your face, arms, and legs.

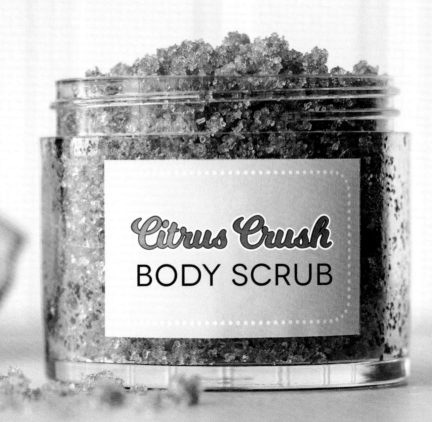

CITRUS CRUSH BODY SCRUB

Inspired by Soap & Glory's Sugar Crush Body Scrub

The brown sugar steals the show in this body scrub. It melts on your skin while it flakes away dry skin.

MAKES 1 (7-OUNCE) BODY SCRUB

2.5 ounces sea salt

2.5 ounces brown sugar

2 ounces almond oil

3–6 drops lemon or lime essential oil

1 (8-ounce) airtight container

HOW TO MAKE:

1 Combine sea salt and brown sugar in a large mixing bowl.

2 Drizzle almond oil on top and stir well until salt and sugar are coated.

3 Add essential oil and stir the mixture well to combine.

4 Scoop the mixture into the airtight container.

HOW TO USE:

1 Use this body scrub once or twice a week on wet skin. Use a clean, dry spoon to scoop 1–2 tablespoons out of the container and take this with you to the shower or bathtub.

2 Gently massage this scrub on wet skin. Rinse it off.

3 Use it last in your shower routine to leave a moisturizing layer on your skin, or lather your body with soap afterward.

4 Oils can make your bathtub or shower floor slippery, so don't forget to clean up after you are done!

HOW TO STORE:

Store in a cool, dry place and keep all water out of the container. This body scrub can keep up to 3 months.

GLIMMER BODY SPRAY

Inspired by Victoria's Secret's PINK Scented Shimmer Mist

It's your time to shine. This quick, spray-on dry oil has extra moisturizing powers, a delightful floral scent, and—of course—sparkles!

MAKES 1 (1.6-OUNCE) BODY SPRAY

1.5 ounces grapeseed oil

1 (2-ounce) spray or pump bottle

10 drops vitamin E oil

3 drops ylang-ylang essential oil

3 drops geranium essential oil

2 teaspoons pearl cosmetic mica

HOW TO MAKE:

1 Pour grapeseed oil into the bottle. Use a small funnel to avoid spilling.

2 Add vitamin E oil and essential oils to the bottle.

3 Add cosmetic mica last. Screw on the top and shake vigorously to combine all ingredients.

HOW TO USE:

1 The oil and glitter will separate, so shake the bottle vigorously before each use.

2 Spray on dry skin and spread the glitter and oil with your hands. Spray this glimmer body oil away from your clothes.

HOW TO STORE:

Store in a cool, dry place out of direct sunlight up to 3 months.

HAND BALM IN A TIN

Inspired by Burt's Bees' Hand Salve

Your hands handle a lot throughout the day. And it starts to show when they feel dry and cracked. This easy recipe uses a kitchen favorite, olive oil, to make a super simple moisturizing balm.

MAKES 1 (1.7-OUNCE) HAND BALM

0.2 ounce beeswax pellets

1.5 ounces olive oil

1 teaspoon kaolin clay

6 drops lavender essential oil

1 (2-ounce) aluminum tin container

HOW TO MAKE:

1 Slowly melt beeswax and olive oil in a double boiler over medium heat. Stir occasionally to combine the ingredients.

2 Add clay to the melted mixture. Stir until the powder has completely dissolved.

3 Take the double boiler off the heat and add essential oil. Stir to make sure all of the ingredients are mixed well.

4 Pour the mixture into the container.

5 Allow to cool 2–3 hours or until the balm has set before use. Place covered in the refrigerator to quicken the cooling process.

HOW TO USE:

1 When your hands can use a little TLC, use clean, dry fingers to remove a little bit of the balm.

2 Use the heat of your hands to melt the balm and massage it into your palms, fingers, and around your nails.

HOW TO STORE:

Store in a cool, dry place and keep all water out of the container. This hand cream can keep up to 3 months.

PINKISH BODY SCRUB

Inspired by Herbivore Botanicals' Coco Rose Body Polish

MAKES 1 (10.5-OUNCE) BODY SCRUB

1 ounce shea butter

1.5 ounces coconut oil

8 ounces sugar

1 teaspoon pink clay

10 drops rose geranium essential oil

1 (11-ounce) airtight container

This scrub gets its natural pink shade from detoxifying clay. Sugar buffs away flaky skin, and shea butter and coconut oil make your skin irresistibly soft. The delicious rose scent is just a bonus.

Price Drop

To make your scrub smell like roses, you need an essential oil. Essential oil made from roses, also known as rosa damascena essential oil, can be very pricey. That's why I like to use rose geranium essential oil instead. Your scrub smells equally amazing for a fraction of the cost.

HOW TO MAKE:

1 Melt shea butter and coconut oil in a double boiler over medium heat. Stir the mixture occasionally.

2 Take the double boiler off the heat and stir in sugar and pink clay.

3 Add essential oil and stir until all the ingredients are well combined. Scoop into the container and let sit 1–2 hours before use.

HOW TO USE:

1 Use clean hands or a spoon or spatula to scoop 1–2 tablespoons of scrub out of the container.

2 Gently massage the scrub on wet skin. Use 1–2 times a week. Rinse with water.

3 Wash with soap after you use this scrub if you don't like the moisturizing layer left on your skin. Oils can make your bathtub or shower floor slippery, so don't forget to clean up after you are done!

HOW TO STORE:

Store in a cool, dry place and keep all water out of the container. This body scrub can keep up to 3 months.

MINTY FEET MASK

Inspired by The Body Shop's Peppermint Intensive Cooling Foot Rescue

This mint-infused treatment is your best bet for tired feet. Tingly peppermint freshens those toes, while the moisturizing butters and oils work to soften rough spots and cracked heels.

MAKES 1 (4-OUNCE) BALM

0.2 ounce beeswax pellets

0.3 ounce cocoa butter

3.5 ounces olive oil

15 drops peppermint essential oil

1 (4.5-ounce) airtight container

HOW TO MAKE:

1 Slowly melt beeswax, cocoa butter, and olive oil in a double boiler over medium heat. Stir occasionally until the ingredients have melted.

2 Take the double boiler off the heat as soon as the mixture has melted. Let the mixture cool a little and then add essential oil.

3 Stir well to make sure all ingredients are blended together and pour the mixture into the container. Allow to cool and set 2–3 hours before use.

HOW TO USE:

1 Using a cotton pad apply a thin layer all over your feet or target specific areas.

2 Put on some socks and sleep on it. Wake up with a pair of brand-new feet!

3 Wash your hands after using this product, and don't use this mask on blisters or open wounds!

HOW TO STORE:

Store in a cool, dry place out of direct sunlight and keep all water out of the container. This feet mask can keep up to 6 months.

NATURAL TAN LOTION

Inspired by Soap & Glory's The Righteous Butter Instant Sunkissed Tint Body Lotion

MAKES 1 (5.6-OUNCE) BODY BALM

1.6 ounces mango butter

1.8 ounces coconut oil

1.8 ounces coffee-infused grapeseed oil (see sidebar on page 134)

30 drops vitamin E oil

1–2 tablespoons cocoa powder

1 teaspoon gold cosmetic mica (optional)

2 (100-milliliter) soft tube containers

Coffee-infused oil and cocoa powder each give your skin a natural bronze tint. Add a drop or two of vanilla essential oil to the mix and you have the best-smelling lotion in the world! Cocoa powder gives you the ultimate all-natural experience, but if you want a more traditional lotion, swap it for a few teaspoons of bronze cosmetic mica.

HOW TO MAKE:

1 Melt mango butter in a double boiler over medium heat. Or melt mango butter in a heat-proof container in the microwave on a low setting (650 watts or lower) using 1-minute intervals. Stir mango butter between intervals until it's completely melted.

2 Pour melted mango butter into a large mixing bowl. Add coconut oil and coffee-infused grapeseed oil. Stir the ingredients until they have all melted together.

3 Set the mixing bowl aside or place it covered in the refrigerator for about 50 minutes until the mixture starts to thicken.

4 Add vitamin E oil, cocoa powder, and cosmetic mica (if using) to the mixture. Carefully whip the mixture using an electric whisk or mixer on a low setting. The mixture is ready once it has a creamy, fluffy consistency.

5 Divide the mixture between the tubes.

Continued on page 134 ▶

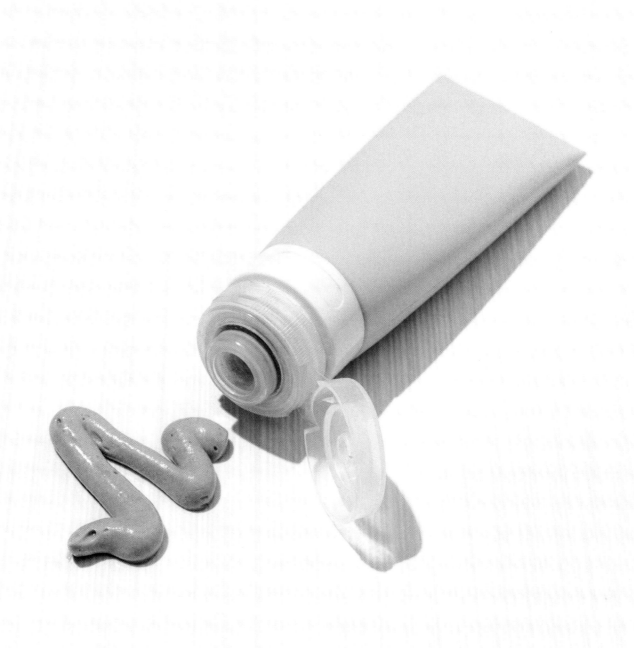

How to Make Coffee-Infused Grapeseed Oil

To make your own coffee-infused grapeseed oil: Infuse ½ cup grapeseed oil with ¼ cup dry ground coffee beans using the cold infusion method described at the beginning of this chapter. Store any leftover oil in an air-tight container up to 3 months. You can also use this oil to make the You're Golden Eye Mask in Chapter 2.

HOW TO USE:

1. Apply a very small amount of the lotion on any body part visible to the eye and in need of a tint. Gently massage it into your skin until there are no more streaks. Avoid places where the lotion can gather, like the insides of your elbows and knees.

2. Give the lotion a few minutes to air-dry.

HOW TO STORE:

Store in a cool, dry place up to 3 months.

SHINY BODY OIL

Inspired by Nars' Monoï Body Glow II

Tahitian monoï oil is made by infusing coconut oil with lovely-smelling tiaré flowers. The manufacturing process of authentic monoï oil has to follow strict guidelines and makes the final product expensive. Instead of using monoï oil, we are making our own vanilla, floral-scented body oil.

MAKES 1 (4-OUNCE) BODY OIL

4 ounces vanilla-infused coconut oil (see sidebar)

3–6 drops ylang-ylang essential oil

1 (5-ounce) airtight container

HOW TO MAKE:

1 Melt vanilla-infused coconut oil in a double boiler over medium heat. Or melt coconut oil in a heatproof container in the microwave (650 watts or lower) for 1 minute.

2 Take the double boiler off the heat or take the container out of the microwave. Add essential oil and stir to combine.

3 Pour the mixture into the airtight container. If coconut oil is liquid at room temperature where you live, you can use a flip-cap or pump bottle.

HOW TO USE:

1 Scoop or pour about ½ tablespoon oil into the palm of your hand.

2 Spread it out evenly on clean, dry skin. Give the oil some time to sink in before putting on your clothes.

HOW TO STORE:

Store in a cool, dry place out of direct sunlight up to 6 months.

How to Make Vanilla-Infused Coconut Oil

You will need one vanilla bean and about 4 ounces of coconut oil to make your own vanilla-infused oil. Cut the vanilla bean into ½" pieces, place them in a double boiler, and scoop coconut oil on top. Use the hot infusion method described earlier in this chapter to infuse the coconut oil with the vanilla. Strain the oil following the instructions until it's clear. Store in an airtight container for up to 6 months.

SAVE YOUR SOLES SPRAY

Inspired by Earth Therapeutics' Tea Tree Oil Foot Spray

MAKES 1 (2-OUNCE) SPRAY

1 teaspoon vegetable glycerin

3 drops tea tree essential oil

1 drop peppermint essential oil (optional)

¼ cup witch hazel

1 (2.5-ounce) spray bottle

Your poor feet. They literally carry your body from one place to the next. Give those soles some love with this refreshing spray.

HOW TO MAKE:

1 Scoop glycerin into a small mixing bowl.

2 Carefully add essential oils and stir to mix.

3 Use a small funnel to pour witch hazel into the spray bottle.

4 Add the glycerin mixture to the bottle. Screw on the top and shake until all the ingredients are combined.

HOW TO USE:

Shake the bottle before each use to mix the water and essential oils. Spray lightly on tired feet in need of refreshment. Repeat as often as needed.

HOW TO STORE:

Store in the refrigerator and use within 3–5 days.

SUPER SALVE

Inspired by Yes To's Coconut Head-to-Toe Restoring Balm

What if you could make a balm that does it all? This Super Salve is just that. Dry ends? Rub a little bit of balm on them. Dry patch of skin? This balm will fix that for you. The star ingredient in this moisturizing Super Salve is the coconut oil. The beeswax makes sure it stays put.

MAKES 1 (1-OUNCE) MOISTURIZING BALM

0.1 ounce beeswax pellets

0.9 ounce coconut oil

1 (1-ounce) airtight container

HOW TO MAKE:

1. Melt beeswax in a double boiler over medium heat.

2. Add coconut oil to the double boiler as soon as the beeswax starts to melt.

3. Stir the melted mixture to make sure the ingredients are well combined and pour into the container.

HOW TO USE:

1. Scoop a small amount of the product out of the container with clean, dry fingers.

2. Apply the balm on any dry areas and massage it in with your fingertips.

3. Give the balm a few seconds to sink in.

HOW TO STORE:

Store in a cool, dry place out of direct sunlight up to 6 months.

SPARKLE SCRUB

Inspired by Frank Body's Shimmer Scrub

MAKES 1 (8.2-OUNCE) BODY SCRUB

2 ounces sugar

2.5 ounces salt

2 ounces ground coffee beans

1.7 ounces grapeseed oil

10 drops vitamin E oil

1 tablespoon biodegradable glitter or gold/pearl cosmetic mica

1 (10-ounce) airtight container

Add a little sparkle and a dose of caffeine to your morning shower routine! This scrub is made with salt and can sting open wounds. If you have cuts or scrapes, you can make this with more sugar or ground coffee beans instead of the salt.

HOW TO MAKE:

1 Combine sugar, salt, and ground coffee beans in a medium mixing bowl.

2 Stir in grapeseed oil and add vitamin E oil.

3 Add biodegradable glitter or cosmetic mica and stir the mixture well to combine all the ingredients.

4 Scoop body scrub into the airtight container.

HOW TO USE:

1 Use clean, dry hands or a spoon to scoop 1–2 tablespoons of the product out of the container before you hop into the shower or bath.

2 Gently massage the scrub on wet skin. Use this scrub 1 or 2 times a week. Rinse to reveal silky smooth, sparkling skin.

3 Oils can make your bathtub or shower floor slippery, so don't forget to clean up after you are done!

HOW TO STORE:

Store in a cool, dry place and keep all water out of the container. This body scrub can keep up to 3 months.

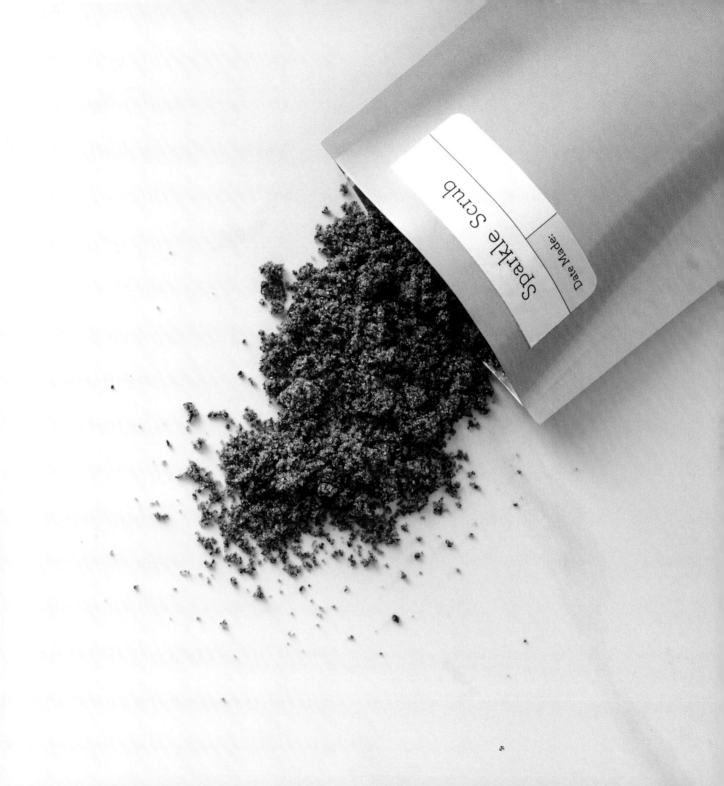

SUGARCOAL BODY SCRUB

Inspired by Origins' Clear Improvement Detoxifying Charcoal Body Scrub

MAKES 1 (6-OUNCE) BODY SCRUB

2 ounces sea salt

2 ounces brown sugar

1 teaspoon activated charcoal powder

1.5 ounces olive oil

1 (7-ounce) airtight container

This pitch-black sugar scrub exfoliates, while the activated charcoal powder absorbs impurities.

HOW TO MAKE:

1. Combine sea salt, brown sugar, and activated charcoal powder in a large mixing bowl. Stir well.

2. Drizzle olive oil on top. Stir until the dry ingredients are coated evenly.

3. Scoop the body scrub into the airtight container.

HOW TO USE:

1. Use this body scrub once or twice a week on wet skin. Scoop 1–2 tablespoons out of the container using a spoon or clean, dry fingers. Take this with you into the shower or bathtub.

2. Gently massage the scrub into your skin. Rinse it off.

3. Use soap to wash off any residue. Oils can make your bathtub or shower floor slippery and the activated charcoal can be messy, so don't forget to clean up after you are done!

HOW TO STORE:

Store in a cool, dry place and keep all water out of the container. This body scrub can keep up to 6 months.

FOAM-UP BODY SCRUB

Inspired by Victoria's Secret's Smoothie Wash

This body scrub foams up as you apply it. Use this scrub right before you shave your legs for the ultimate pampering experience!

MAKES 1 (13-OUNCE) FOAMING BODY SCRUB

8 ounces sugar

4 ounces coconut oil

1 ounce unscented liquid Castile soap

15 drops essential oil of your choice

1 (15-ounce) container

HOW TO MAKE:

1 Add sugar, coconut oil, Castile soap, and essential oil to a large mixing bowl.

2 Use an electric whisk or mixer to whip the ingredients together. Start at the lowest setting. Keep whipping the mixture until all the ingredients are combined.

3 Scoop the mixture into the airtight container.

HOW TO USE:

1 Before heading to the shower or bathtub scoop 1–2 tablespoons out of the container and take it with you.

2 Gently rub the scrub over wet skin. Rinse off with plenty of water. Use this scrub once or twice a week. Oils can make your bathtub or shower floor slippery, so don't forget to clean up after you are done!

HOW TO STORE:

Store in a cool, dry place and keep all water out of the container. This body scrub can keep up to 3 months.

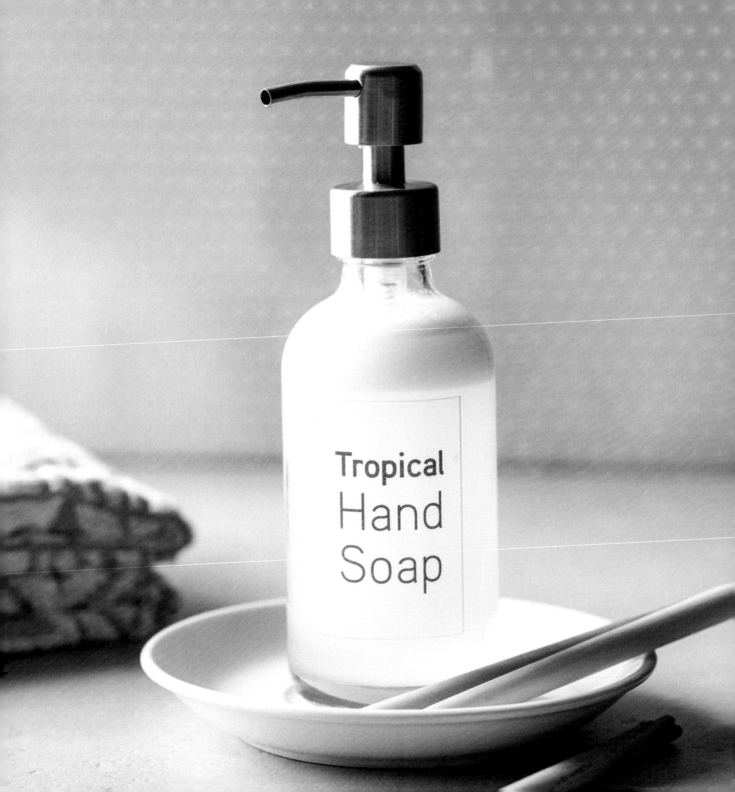

TROPICAL HAND SOAP

Inspired by Yes To's Coconut Lemongrass Liquid Hand Soap

You'll feel like you're on a tropical island when you wash up with this all-natural liquid soap. Palm trees, coconut shells everywhere, a citrusy breeze in the air—oh wait; yup, you're still standing in your bathroom.

MAKES 1 (2.5-OUNCE) LIQUID HAND SOAP

2 ounces unscented liquid Castile soap

1 (3-ounce) airtight pump bottle

½ tablespoon glycerin

1 tablespoon fractionated coconut oil

6 drops lemongrass essential oil

HOW TO MAKE:

1 Use a small funnel to pour Castile soap into the pump bottle.

2 Add glycerin, fractionated coconut oil, and lemongrass essential oil.

3 Take the funnel out of the bottle and screw the pump top back on. Shake to combine all the ingredients.

HOW TO USE:

Wet your hands first. Add one pump of liquid soap and rub your hands together to create a lather. Wash your hands as you normally would. Rinse off with plenty of water.

HOW TO STORE:

This hand soap can keep up to 6 months in an airtight container.

Fractionated Coconut Oil

In most cases I'll recommend you to go with the unrefined version of an oil. And I do love my tub of solid extra-virgin coconut oil. But its refined counterpart has its benefits too; for example, fractionated coconut oil stays liquid at room temperature. You can easily substitute the fractionated coconut oil in this recipe with another carrier oil, like olive or sweet almond oil.

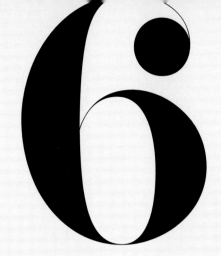

CHAPTER 6
BATH FUN

Bath products are great projects if you're new to DIY beauty. Don't let the ingredients lists or steps of these recipes scare you. Making your own bath products is such an addictive activity. There really are no limits to your creativity. You can play around with different colors, shapes, scents, and textures as much as you please.

DIY bath products also make the best homemade gifts. You can make a pink or blue bath bomb for a baby shower, a bath melt shaped like a Christmas tree, or a scented bath oil for that one friend who loves the scent of lavender so much. Wrap your customized creation in some cute handmade packaging and add a sweet handwritten note. Your gift is sure to melt the heart of whoever receives it. And of course you have to make a couple of extra bath products to keep for yourself!

THE PERFECT BOMB

There's no more satisfying feeling in the world than creating your own bath bomb—except watching it turn into a fizz party in your bathtub. The science behind a bath bomb is actually very simple. If you combine citric acid with baking soda and a large amount of water, it starts to fizz like a firecracker.

As much as bath bombs are probably my favorite science project, they are not an exact science. Different factors can play a role in the making process. Follow these bath bomb guidelines, and your bath bombs will always be a success.

- **Stick to a recipe you know works.** The ratio I like to use for my bath bombs is one part citric acid powder for every two parts baking soda. You can also add one part cornstarch or arrowroot powder to your recipe. This will make the mixture less likely to fizz during the liquid phase of the recipe (a great hack for first-time bath bomb makers).

- **Be careful when adding your liquid.** The liquid phase is when bath bomb making starts to get complicated. By adding a small amount of liquid, you make sure the mixture sticks together. But you don't want to add too much, or you'll get a fizz party in your mixing bowl. There's no exact number when it comes to the amount of liquid you need. It depends, for example, on the humidity in the room based on the weather conditions and the time of year. Using a spray bottle is the best way to avoid adding too much liquid at once. Whisk well in between sprays and check regularly to see if the mixture clumps together. You can check if the mixture is ready by taking a handful in the palm of you hand. Make a fist and release. If the mixture sticks together, it's ready. If it falls apart, you need to add a little bit more liquid.

- **Add some oil first.** Not only will this release a great moisturizing oil into your bathwater, but the oil will also help the mixture stick together, so you'll need less liquid. My favorite oils for bath bombs are olive oil, sweet almond oil, and coconut oil.

- **Give it time to dry.** You've created your epic bath bomb. Now it's time to reveal it and use it, right? Not so fast. The mixture needs time to dry. An hour or two should do the trick, but I recommend leaving your bath bombs in their molds overnight just to be sure.

OUT OF THIS WORLD BATH BOMB

Inspired by Lush's Intergalactic Bath Bomb

Let this bath bomb take you on a journey far, far away!

MAKES 1 GIANT BATH BOMB OR 3 MEDIUM-SIZED BATH BOMBS

$\frac{1}{2}$ cup baking soda

$\frac{1}{4}$ cup citric acid

$\frac{1}{4}$ cup cornstarch

12 drops essential oil of your choice

1 tablespoon sweet almond oil

Different shades of coloring (cosmetic mica, soap coloring, or food coloring)

Witch hazel (as needed)

1 tablespoon sprinkles of your choice

Round bath bomb molds

HOW TO MAKE:

1 Combine baking soda, citric acid, and cornstarch in a large mixing bowl. Mix well with a whisk or spoon to blend the ingredients.

2 Carefully add essential oil and almond oil while you keep stirring the mixture.

3 Divide the mixture between several smaller mixing bowls. Add a different color to each batch—blue, yellow, purple, or red. Use different colors and create your own interpretation of a clear night sky. Start small and keep adding more color until the mixture has the desired color.

4 If you use a liquid coloring, you might not need to add more liquid. Otherwise, add a little witch hazel to each batch until the mixture starts to clump together in the palm of your hand.

5 Add sprinkles of your choice to one or more of the batches.

6 Start layering different colors in both sides of your molds. When they are overflowing press both sides together.

7 Let the bath bombs dry in their molds overnight.

Continued on page 148 ▸

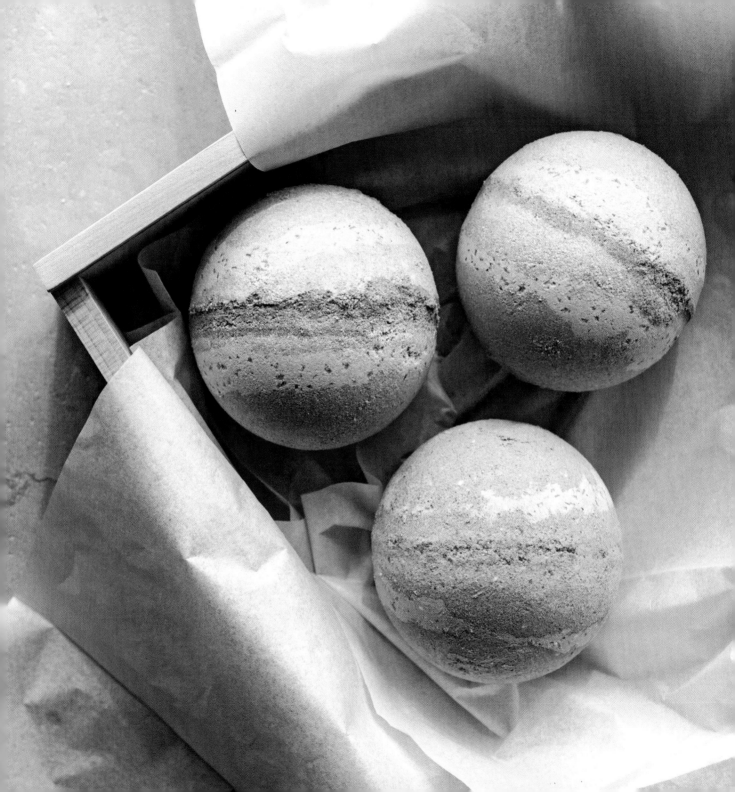

Switch Out the Sugar

Not crazy about sugar sprinkles in your bath bomb? Use jojoba beads, cosmetic mica, or edible glitter luster dust instead. You can buy jojoba beads online and find edible glitter luster dust in the baking section at your local grocery store.

HOW TO USE:

Drop a bath bomb in your bathtub and forget about the world outside for a moment. Watch as it fizzes away and turns your bathwater into a star-studded Milky Way.

HOW TO STORE:

Store bath bombs in a cool, dry place. You can wrap them individually in tissue paper or a similar material and store them all together in a container with a lid. They can also be stored individually in paper or plastic bags as long as they seal well. Bath bombs are best used within 6 months for optimal fizz.

BATH CANDIES

Inspired by Lush's Bath Oils

This guilt-free indulgence will make your skin feel silky soft! You can also kick these candies up a notch by rolling them in Epsom salt, pink Himalayan salt, or dried flower petals to coat the outside. Or get creative with jojoba beads or biodegradable glitter!

MAKES 2.4-OUNCES OR ABOUT 5 BATH CANDIES

1.2 ounces cocoa butter

0.6 ounce coconut oil

0.6 ounce jojoba oil

1 teaspoon pink cosmetic mica

10 drops essential oil of your choice

1 tablespoon silver cosmetic mica

HOW TO MAKE:

1. Melt cocoa butter in a double boiler over medium heat. Or melt cocoa butter in a heat-proof container in the microwave on a low setting (650 watts or lower) using 1-minute intervals. Stir between intervals until cocoa butter has turned liquid.

2. Pour melted cocoa butter into a mixing bowl and stir in coconut oil and jojoba oil.

3. Color the mixture with pink cosmetic mica. Stir well until the color is distributed evenly.

4. Add up to 10 drops essential oil depending on your preference and skin sensitivity. Stir to combine.

5. Wait for the mixture to solidify. You can cover the bowl and set it in the refrigerator for about 1 hour to speed up the process.

6. Use a teaspoon or melon baller to form little balls from the mixture. Roll them between your hands to help create a round shape.

7. Roll the balls in silver cosmetic mica or another color of your choice to coat the outsides.

HOW TO USE:

Drop one bath candy in a bathtub filled with warm water. Let it melt away in the water. The oils in this product can make your bathtub slippery, so don't forget to clean up after you are done!

HOW TO STORE:

These beauties can melt if you live in a warm climate. If this happens, store them in an airtight container in the refrigerator. These bath candies can keep up to 6 months.

PIÑATA BATH BOMB

Inspired by Lush's Sakura Bath Bomb

1/4 cup Epsom salt

4 liquid colorings of your choice

1/2 cup baking soda

1/4 cup citric acid

1/4 cup cornstarch

1 tablespoon sweet almond oil

10 drops essential oil of your choice

Witch hazel (as needed)

Round bath bomb molds

No candy is hiding inside this piñata. Instead, this bath bomb holds lovely, soothing bath salts.

HOW TO MAKE:

1 Divide Epsom salt between four mixing bowls. Add a different color to each batch and let the salt soak up the dye. Start with 1 drop. If the colors are not showing enough, you can add one or two more drops. Set aside the salt to dry.

2 Combine baking soda, citric acid, and cornstarch in a large mixing bowl. Mix well with a whisk or spoon to blend the ingredients.

3 Carefully add almond oil and essential oil to the dry ingredients and continue stirring the mixture.

4 Slowly add small amounts of witch hazel until the mixture starts to clump together in the palm of your hand. You usually need between 1 teaspoon and 1 tablespoon.

5 Scoop 1/3 teaspoon salt from each bowl into your round molds. These will sit on top when you reveal your bath bomb.

6 Add the rest of the salt to the bath bomb mixture. Stir gently to mix the salt with the other ingredients.

7 Scoop the mixture into the molds. Fill them up until they are overflowing, then push both sides together.

8 Let the bath bombs dry in their molds overnight.

HOW TO USE:

Draw a bath and get ready for action. Drop the bath bomb into your bathwater and let it crack open to reveal its beautiful contents: colorful Epsom salt confetti.

HOW TO STORE:

Store bath bombs in a cool, dry place. You can wrap them individually in tissue paper or a similar material and store them all together in a container with a lid. They can also be stored individually in paper or plastic bags as long as they seal well. Bath bombs are best used within 6 months for optimal fizz.

BLUSH SOAP BAR

Inspired by Herbivore Botanicals' Pink Clay Gentle Cleanse Clay Soap Bar

MAKES 1 (4.3-OUNCE) SOAP BAR

4 ounces white melt-and-pour soap base

1 tablespoon coconut oil

$\frac{1}{2}$ teaspoon pink clay

8 drops geranium essential oil

8 drops orange essential oil

1 soap mold

Soap Goals

Melt-and-pour soap base: the name gives it away. This easy premade base allows you to simply melt and pour your own soaps. The quality of your home-made soaps will of course de-pend on the quality of your base. Make sure to get a natural melt-and-pour soap base.

This floral soap bar gets its beautiful natural color from pink clay.

HOW TO MAKE:

1 Cut melt-and-pour soap base into $\frac{1}{2}$" cubes.

2 Melt cubes in a double boiler over medium heat. Or melt cubes in a heatproof bowl in the microwave on a low setting (650 watts or lower). Stir every 30 seconds until cubes have melted.

3 Take the double boiler off the heat or take the bowl out of the microwave. Add the coco-nut oil and stir until the oil has dissolved.

4 Add pink clay and stir until the mixture has an even pink color.

5 Add essential oils and stir to distribute the drops evenly.

6 Pour the melted mixture into the soap mold. Wait 1–2 hours for the bar to cool down.

HOW TO USE:

Wet the soap bar and rub on wet skin. Rub between your hands to create more of a lather.

HOW TO STORE:

Let the soap air-dry after each use. Use this soap bar within 6 months.

LOLLY BOMBS

Inspired by Victoria's Secret's PINK Popsicle Bath Bombs

Bring the summer into your bathroom! No matter what the temperature is outside, these bath bombs will surely brighten your day.

MAKES 3–4 BATH BOMB POPS

½ tablespoon shea butter

½ cup baking soda

¼ cup citric acid

¼ cup cornstarch

15 drops essential oil of your choice

Few drops coloring of your choice (cosmetic mica, soap coloring, or food coloring)

Witch hazel (as needed)

3–4 popsicle molds

Wooden craft sticks

HOW TO MAKE:

1 Melt shea butter in a double boiler over medium heat. Or melt shea butter in a heatproof container in the microwave on a low setting (650 watts or lower) using 1-minute intervals. Stir between intervals until shea butter has melted.

2 Combine baking soda, citric acid, and cornstarch in a large mixing bowl. Mix well with a whisk or spoon to blend the ingredients.

3 Carefully add melted shea butter and essential oil to the dry ingredients and continue stirring the mixture.

4 Add coloring of your choice to the batch until the mixture has the color you want. Divide the mixture among two or three mixing bowls if you want to make an assortment of different colored Lolly Bombs.

5 Slowly add small amounts of witch hazel until the mixture starts to clump together in the palm of your hand. As little as a teaspoon can be enough.

6 Scoop the mixture into the popsicle molds. Press down the mixture firmly when you reach the top.

Continued on page 155 ▸

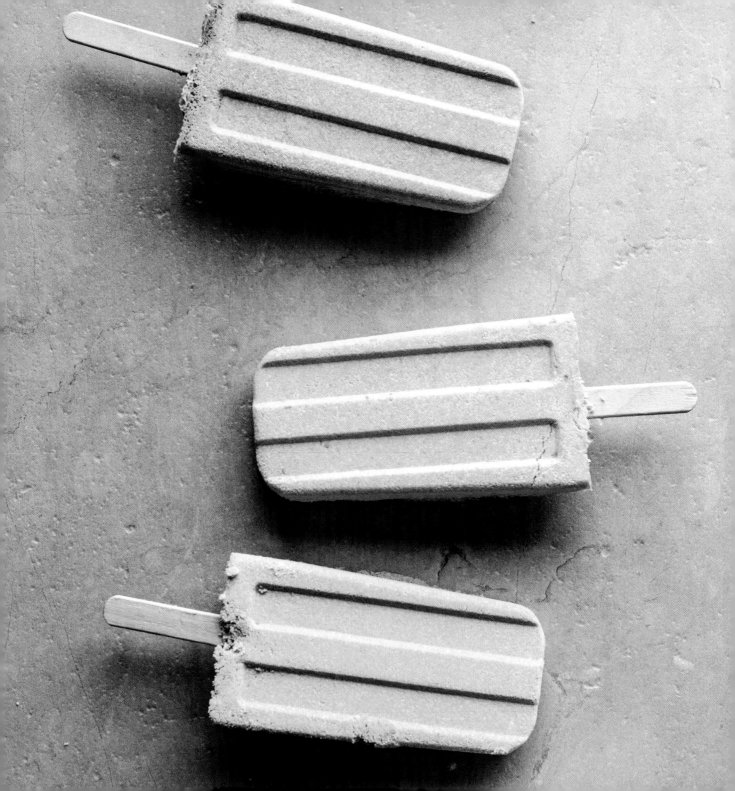

7 Stick a wooden craft stick into the center of each mold. Press down the mixture on each side.

8 Let the bath bombs dry in their molds overnight. Carefully remove them from their molds the next day.

HOW TO USE:

Draw a bath. Drop in a Lolly Bomb and watch it fizz away. Hop into the bathtub and close your eyes.

HOW TO STORE:

Always store bath bombs in a cool, dry place. You can wrap them individually in tissue paper or a similar material and store them all together in a container with a lid. They can also be stored individually in paper or plastic bags as long as they seal well. Bath bombs are best used within 6 months for optimal fizz.

Get Creative

You can also layer different colors on top of each other in these bath bombs or swirl them together. Try adding dried flowers or pretty, colorful jojoba beads to the mix. There really are no limits to your imagination!

I HEART BATH BOMBS

Inspired by Bath & Body Works' Bath Fizzies

Personalize the color and scent of these bath bombs, and you're sure to melt a few hearts (pun totally intended).

MAKES ABOUT 3 HEART-SHAPED BATH BOMBS

½ cup baking soda

¼ cup citric acid

¼ cup cornstarch

¼ cup Epsom salt

1 tablespoon sweet almond oil

15 drops essential oil of your choice

Few drops coloring of your choice (cosmetic mica, soap coloring, or food coloring)

Witch hazel (as needed)

3 heart-shaped molds

Color Correction

You can find soap or bath bomb coloring at a craft store or online. You can also add a few teaspoons of cosmetic mica to your dry ingredients. Or use natural colors, such as turmeric powder for a touch of yellow, matcha for a bright green color, or beetroot powder for a pretty pink color.

HOW TO MAKE:

1 Combine baking soda, citric acid, cornstarch, and Epsom salt in a large mixing bowl. Mix well to blend the ingredients.

2 Carefully add sweet almond oil and essential oil to the dry ingredients and continue stirring.

3 Add coloring to the batch while you keep stirring until the mixture has the color you want.

4 Slowly add small amounts of witch hazel until the mixture starts to clump together in the palm of your hand. As little as a teaspoon can be enough.

5 Scoop the mixture into the heart-shaped molds. Press down the mixture slightly with your fingertips when you have reached the top of the mold.

6 Let the bath bombs dry in their molds overnight.

HOW TO USE:

Drop a heart-shaped bath bomb in your bathwater and watch it fizz away!

HOW TO STORE:

Store bath bombs in a cool, dry place. You can wrap them individually in tissue paper or a similar material and store them all together in a container with a lid. They can also be stored individually in paper or plastic bags as long as they seal well. Bath bombs are best used within 6 months for optimal fizz.

MERBABE BATH BOMB

Inspired by Lush's Big Blue Mind-Clearing Seaweed Soak

You'll feel like a mermaid floating in your seaweed-spiked bathwater.

HOW TO MAKE:

1 Combine baking soda, citric acid, and sea salt in a large mixing bowl. Whisk or stir well.

2 Melt coconut oil using the double boiler method over medium heat. Or melt in a heatproof container in the microwave for 1 minute.

3 Scatter melted coconut oil and essential oil drops over the dry mixture and stir to combine.

4 Divide the mixture into two batches. Add blue coloring to one batch and stir until the mixture is colored evenly.

5 Add 1/2 teaspoon witch hazel to the first batch and stir. Continue until the mixture clumps together in your hand. Repeat with the other batch.

6 Break dried seaweed into smaller pieces using your fingers or the back of a spoon. Add the pieces to the blue batch.

7 Fill one side of each bath bomb mold about halfway with the white mixture. Scoop the blue mixture on top until the mold is overflowing. Do the same for the other half. Press both sides together. Let the bath bombs dry in the molds overnight.

HOW TO USE:

Drop the bath bomb in an ocean, I mean bathtub, filled with water. While the bath bomb fizzes away, the seaweed pieces will start to float on top of the water.

MAKES 1 GIANT BATH BOMB OR 3 MEDIUM-SIZED BATH BOMBS

1/2 cup baking soda

1/4 cup citric acid

1/4 cup coarse sea salt

1 tablespoon coconut oil

12 drops essential oil of your choice

Blue liquid or mica coloring

1 teaspoon witch hazel (as needed)

1 tablespoon dried arame seaweed

Round bath bomb molds

HOW TO STORE:

Store bath bombs in a cool, dry place. You can wrap them individually in tissue paper or a similar material and store them all together in a container with a lid. They can also be stored individually in paper or plastic bags as long as they seal well. Bath bombs are best used within 6 months for optimal fizz.

MILKSHAKE BOMBS

Inspired by Soap & Glory's Fizz-a-Ball Bath Bombs

**MAKES 1 GIANT BATH BOMB OR
3 MEDIUM-SIZED BATH BOMBS**

1/2 cup baking soda

1/4 cup citric acid

1/4 cup cornstarch

1 tablespoon unscented liquid Castile soap

6 drops lime essential oil

Liquid or mica pink and yellow coloring (as needed)

Witch hazel (as needed)

Round bath bomb molds

Let's turn our bath into a milkshake with a Milkshake Bomb! This recipe uses Castile soap to add a frothy, creamy layer on top of your bathwater. Because of the Castile soap the bath bombs might expand and change shape a little as they dry. I think that's part of the charm! If you're a beginner, use flexible silicone molds instead.

HOW TO MAKE:

1 Combine baking soda, citric acid, and cornstarch in a large mixing bowl. Mix well with a whisk or spoon to blend the ingredients.

2 Carefully add Castile soap and lime essential oil to the dry ingredients while you keep stirring the mixture.

3 Divide the mixture into two batches in separate smaller mixing bowls. Carefully add yellow coloring to one batch and pink to the other. Stir to evenly distribute the color.

4 Check if the mixtures in both batches clump together in the palm of your hand. If they don't, add a little bit of witch hazel. Don't make the mixture too wet or your bath bombs will stick to your molds!

Continued on page 160 ▶

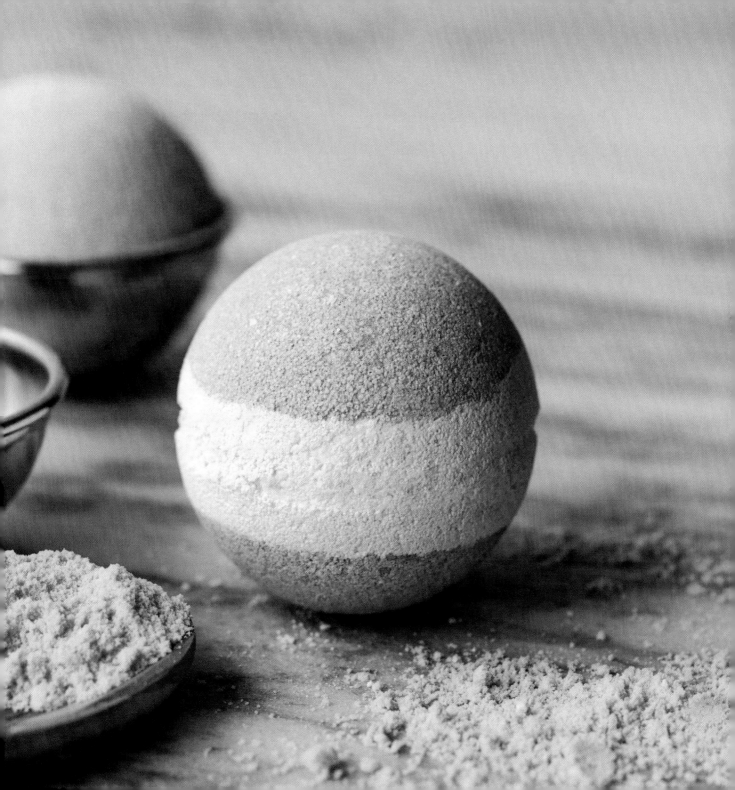

Mix Up Your Milkshake!

The product that inspired these Milkshake Bombs comes in different colors and scents, so feel free to experiment with your own creations. Try rose or vanilla essential oil or whatever other scent relaxes you. And you can go bold or calming with your colors—anything goes!

5 Scoop the pink mixture into the round bath bomb molds, and then layer the yellow color on top until both sides are overflowing. Press both sides of each mold together.

6 Take the bath bombs out of their molds and set aside to dry overnight.

HOW TO USE:

Get the water running in your bath and drop your Milkshake Bomb directly underneath the running tap.

HOW TO STORE:

These bath bombs are best used within 3 months. You can wrap them individually in tissue paper or a similar material and store them all together in a container with a lid. They can also be stored individually in paper or plastic bags as long as they seal well.

PASTEL RAINBOW BATH BOMB

Inspired by Victoria's Secret's PINK Bath Bombs

Make a splash and release a pastel rainbow in your bathtub. The shea butter will moisturize your skin, and the lavender and vanilla oils will delight your senses.

HOW TO MAKE:

1 Melt shea butter in a double boiler over medium heat. Or melt shea butter in a heatproof container in the microwave on a low setting (650 watts or lower) using 1-minute intervals. Stir shea butter between intervals until it's completely melted.

2 Combine baking soda, citric acid, and cornstarch in a large mixing bowl. Mix well with a whisk or spoon to blend the ingredients.

3 Carefully add melted shea butter and essential oils to the dry ingredients while you keep stirring the mixture.

4 Divide the mixture among four mixing bowls.

5 Put about 1 tablespoon witch hazel in a spray bottle. Add 3–6 drops of one coloring to the witch hazel. Spray one of the batches lightly with the colored witch hazel until the mixture clumps together when you squeeze it in the palm of your hand.

MAKES 1 GIANT BATH BOMB OR 3 MEDIUM-SIZED BATH BOMBS

½ tablespoon shea butter

½ cup baking soda

¼ cup citric acid

¼ cup cornstarch

6 drops lavender essential oil

6 drops vanilla essential oil

4 tablespoons witch hazel

Small spray bottle

3-6 drops pink, green, blue, and yellow liquid coloring

Round bath bomb molds

Continued on next page ▸

True Colors

These bath bombs are super adorable sitting next to your bathtub. But because we've diluted the coloring, they won't color your bathwater. If you want your bathwater to change color, I recommend the Out of This World Bath Bomb or the Milkshake Bombs (both recipes in this chapter), as you add a lot more coloring to those. A good-quality soap or bath bomb coloring should never stain your skin; the coloring will be diluted in plenty of water as you use it.

6 Rinse out the spray bottle and repeat the previous step with a different color and a different batch. Continue until you have four batches in different colors.

7 Scoop 1 tablespoon from each batch into a bath bomb mold. Repeat until each half is overflowing. Press both sides together. Continue until all the batches are used up.

8 Let the bath bombs dry in their molds overnight.

HOW TO USE:

Drop one bath bomb in your bathwater to release the shea butter and essential oils.

HOW TO STORE:

Store bath bombs in a cool, dry place. You can wrap them individually in tissue paper or a similar material and store them all together in a container with a lid. They can also be stored individually in paper or plastic bags as long as they seal well. Bath bombs are best used within 6 months for optimal fizz.

SNOOZE BATH SALTS

Inspired by Bath & Body Works' Sleep: Lavender + Cedarwood Bath Soak

These bath salts don't just look pretty next to your bathtub. The lavender and cedarwood blend will relax your mind, and the salts and baking soda will soothe any aches.

MAKES 11 OUNCES BATH SALTS

1 cup Epsom salt

½ cup baking soda

10 drops lavender essential oil

10 drops cedarwood essential oil

1 (15-ounce) airtight container

HOW TO MAKE:

1 Combine Epsom salt and baking soda in a medium mixing bowl and stir.

2 Disperse essential oils evenly over the mixture. Pour the bath salt mixture into the airtight container. Put on the lid and shake the container to mix the ingredients well.

HOW TO USE:

When you're running a bath, scatter 2–3 tablespoons Snooze Bath Salts under the running tap. Let the salts melt away and the aromas fill your bathroom. Then just sit back and relax.

HOW TO STORE:

Store in an airtight container in a cool, dry place up to 6 months. Keep any water out of the container.

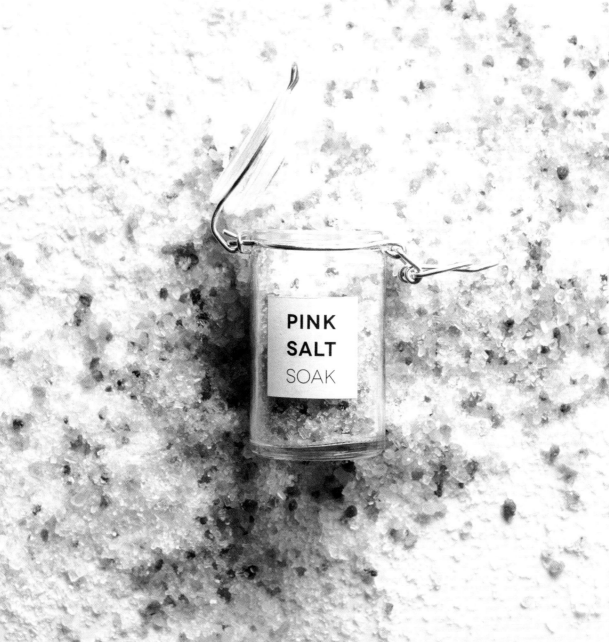

PINK SALT SOAK

Inspired by Herbivore Botanicals' Calm Soaking Salts

This Pink Salt Soak is so easy to make that it's the perfect handmade gift. Score extra creativity points and package it in a pretty glass jar. Decorate the outside with washi tape, tie a cute label around the lid with an equally cute ribbon, and include a personal message.

MAKES 14 OUNCES BATH SOAK

1 cup Epsom salt

½ cup pink Himalayan coarse salt

5 drops ylang-ylang essential oil

10 drops vanilla essential oil

1 (15-ounce) airtight container

HOW TO MAKE:

1 Combine Epsom salt and pink Himalayan salt in a medium mixing bowl.

2 Disperse essential oils evenly over the salts.

3 Transfer the salts into the airtight container. Put on the lid and shake the container to mix the ingredients well.

HOW TO USE:

When you're ready to take a bath, scatter 2–3 tablespoons Pink Salt Soak under the running tap. Let the salts melt away as you sit back and relax.

HOW TO STORE:

Store in an airtight container in a cool, dry place up to 6 months. Keep any water out of the container.

SOAK OIL

Inspired by Burt's Bees' Lemon & Vitamin E Bath & Body Oil

MAKES 1 (4-OUNCE) BATH OIL

1 (4-ounce) pump or flip-cap bottle

4 ounces sweet almond oil

25 drops vitamin E oil

10 drops lemon essential oil

This nourishing soak oil fills your bathroom with an uplifting and refreshing lemon scent!

HOW TO MAKE:

1 Insert a small funnel into the bottle. Carefully pour sweet almond oil into the bottle. Remove the funnel and add vitamin E oil and lemon essential oil.

2 Screw the cap or dispenser back onto the bottle. Shake the bottle to make sure all ingredients are evenly combined.

HOW TO USE:

Add 1–2 tablespoons to your bathwater. Swirl around with your hands to distribute. Oils can make your bathtub slippery, so don't forget to clean up when you are done!

HOW TO STORE:

Store this oil in a cool, dry place and keep all water out of the container. This bath oil can keep up to 6 months.

COUNTRY MASSAGE OIL

Inspired by The Body Shop's Spa of the World French Lavender Massage Oil

This relaxing massage oil smells like the French countryside. Close your eyes and picture a purple field of blossoming lavender flowers!

MAKES 1 (3.5-OUNCE) MASSAGE OIL

3.5 ounces grapeseed oil

20 drops vitamin E oil

1 (4-ounce) pump or flip-cap bottle

15 drops lavender essential oil

HOW TO MAKE:

1 Pour grapeseed oil and vitamin E oil into the bottle. Use a small funnel to avoid spilling.

2 Take the funnel out of the bottle and add essential oil. Screw the top back on and shake until the essential oils are evenly distributed.

HOW TO USE:

1 Take about 1 teaspoon Country Massage Oil in the palm of your hand. Carefully rub your hands together to heat up the oil.

2 Spread the oil evenly over your (or someone else's) body and use it to massage any sore or tight muscles.

HOW TO STORE:

Store in a cool, dry place out of direct sunlight up to 3 months.

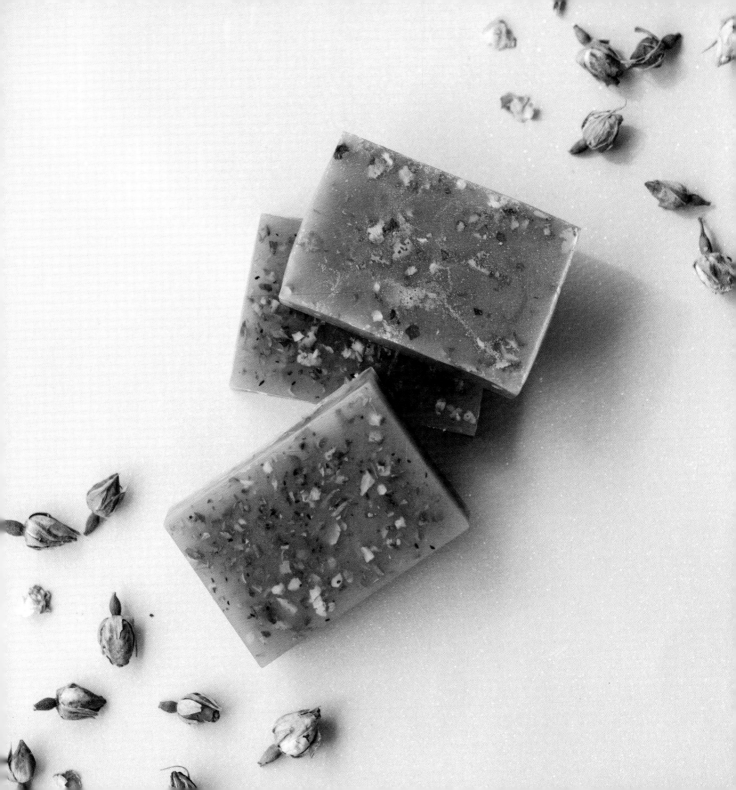

SCRUB AND SUDS BAR

Inspired by The Body Shop's British Rose Exfoliating Soap

This cute petal-specked soap gently cleanses and exfoliates your skin.

HOW TO MAKE:

1 Scoop dried rose petals onto a shallow dish or plate. Crush the petals with the back of a spoon. Add glycerin and stir until the dried flower chunks are evenly coated. Set aside.

2 Cut melt-and-pour soap base into ½" cubes. Place the cubes in a double boiler over medium heat and melt until liquid. Or melt cubes in a heatproof bowl in the microwave on a low setting (650 watts or lower). Stir every 30 seconds until cubes have melted.

3 Once soap base has melted, add shea butter to the double boiler.

4 Add drop of liquid coloring or pinch of mica. Stir until the mixture has turned liquid and the color is distributed evenly.

5 Take the double boiler off the heat and let cool for a few minutes. Carefully stir in the glycerin and flower petal mixture.

6 Add essential oil and stir until it is evenly distributed in the mixture.

7 Pour the soap mixture into the soap mold. Let set 1–2 hours before taking it out of the mold.

HOW TO USE:

Gently rub the soap bar on wet skin. Let the bar air-dry after each use.

MAKES 1 (4.3-OUNCE) SOAP BAR

1 tablespoon dried rose petals

1 teaspoon glycerin

4 ounces clear melt-and-pour soap base

½ tablespoon shea butter

1 drop red or pink liquid soap coloring (or 1 teaspoon cosmetic mica)

15 drops geranium essential oil

1 silicone soap mold

HOW TO STORE:

This Scrub and Suds Bar can keep up to 6 months (but the petals might turn brown after a while) in an airtight container. Let the soap bar air-dry after each use (on a soap tray, for example). If you would like to give this bar as a gift, you can wrap the dry soap bar in craft wrapping paper.

SHOWER TABS

Inspired by Bath & Body Works' Shower Steamers

MAKES ABOUT 10 SHOWER TABS

1 cup baking soda

¹/₂ cup cream of tartar

15–30 drops essential oil of your choice

Witch hazel (as needed)

Silicone ice cube mold

Essential Blends

Pick the right essential oils for your mood. Want a relaxing shower or bath? Go for lavender and cedarwood. Feeling a little under the weather? Use a few drops of eucalyptus and sandalwood. If it's energy and focus you're looking for, try lemongrass and rosemary. Always start with just a few drops, as essential oils can be very overpowering!

These are like bath bombs but for your shower! They're an easy way to bring the relaxing scents of essential oils into your morning or evening shower routine. Vary the amount of essential oil you use based on your scent preferences.

HOW TO MAKE:

1. Combine baking soda and cream of tartar in a large mixing bowl. Stir until you get an even mixture.

2. Carefully add essential oil. Stir the mixture between each drop.

3. Add witch hazel to the mixture. Start with 1 teaspoon. Stir the mixture while you add the witch hazel. Check if the mixture clumps together by taking some in the palm of your hand and squeezing it. If the mixture holds together, it's ready. If it crumbles into a powder, add more witch hazel until it sticks together.

4. Divide the mixture evenly between the molds. Leave the tabs in their molds to dry overnight. Pop them out of their molds and store them in an airtight container until you're ready to use them.

HOW TO USE:

Place one Shower Tab near your shower drain. Shower as you normally would. The warm water will activate the tab, making it fizz away and making the lovely essential oils spread in your shower.

HOW TO STORE:

Store in an airtight container and use within 3 months.

BATH POWDER

Inspired by Aveeno's Soothing Bath Treatment

Want to beat that itch? Bathe in an oatmeal milk bath to help relieve eczema, insect bites, or even a sunburn.

MAKES 2 CUPS BATH POWDER (ABOUT 8 APPLICATIONS)

$2\frac{1}{2}$ cups old-fashioned rolled oats

1 (8-ounce) airtight container

HOW TO MAKE:

1 Blend the oats in a clean, dry food processor or coffee grinder until they turn into a very fine powder. Sift the powder through a fine-mesh sieve if you want to keep only the very fine powder.

2 Transfer oat powder to the airtight container.

HOW TO USE:

1 Draw a bath with lukewarm water. Scatter about $\frac{1}{4}$ cup bath powder in the water.

2 Soak in the water 10–15 minutes.

3 Rinse off and gently pat your skin dry with a towel. Follow with a moisturizing balm.

HOW TO STORE:

Store in a cool, dry place and keep all water out of the container or you'll end up with oat milk that will spoil really fast. This bath powder can keep up to 6 months.

US/METRIC CONVERSION CHART

VOLUME CONVERSIONS

US Volume Measure	Metric Equivalent
⅛ teaspoon	0.5 milliliter
¼ teaspoon	1 milliliter
½ teaspoon	2 milliliters
1 teaspoon	5 milliliters
½ tablespoon	7 milliliters
1 tablespoon (3 teaspoons)	15 milliliters
2 tablespoons (1 fluid ounce)	30 milliliters
¼ cup (4 tablespoons)	60 milliliters
⅓ cup	90 milliliters
½ cup (4 fluid ounces)	125 milliliters
⅔ cup	160 milliliters
¾ cup (6 fluid ounces)	180 milliliters
1 cup (16 tablespoons)	250 milliliters
1 pint (2 cups)	500 milliliters
1 quart (4 cups)	1 liter (about)

WEIGHT CONVERSIONS

US Weight Measure	Metric Equivalent
½ ounce	15 grams
1 ounce	30 grams
2 ounces	60 grams
3 ounces	85 grams
¼ pound (4 ounces)	115 grams
½ pound (8 ounces)	225 grams
¾ pound (12 ounces)	340 grams
1 pound (16 ounces)	454 grams

INDEX